WALKING YOUR WAY TO WEIGHT LOSS PLUS INTERMITTENT FASTING FOR WOMEN

THE ULTIMATE 2 IN 1 COLLECTION FOR UNLOCKING THE SECRETS TO SUSTAINABLE, LONG-TERM WEIGHT LOSS AND A HEALTHY LIFESTYLE

HEALTHFIT PUBLISHING

© **Copyright 2022 - All rights reserved.**

The content contained within this book may not be reproduced, duplicated, or transmitted without direct written permission from the author or the publisher.

Under no circumstances will any blame or legal responsibility be held against the publisher, or author, for any damages, reparation, or monetary loss due to the information contained within this book, either directly or indirectly.

Legal Notice:

This book is copyright protected. It is only for personal use. You cannot amend, distribute, sell, use, quote, or paraphrase any part, or the content within this book, without the consent of the author or publisher.

Disclaimer Notice:

Please note the information contained within this document is for educational and entertainment purposes only. All effort has been executed to present accurate, up-to-date, reliable, complete information. No warranties of any kind are declared or implied. Readers acknowledge that the author is not engaged in the rendering of legal, financial, medical, or professional advice. The content within this book has been derived from various sources. Please consult a licensed professional before attempting any techniques outlined in this book.

By reading this document, the reader agrees that under no circumstances is the author responsible for any losses, direct or indirect, that are incurred as a result of the use of the information contained within this document, including, but not limited to, errors, omissions, or inaccuracies.

CONTENTS

WALKING YOUR WAY TO WEIGHT LOSS
Healthfit Publishing

Introduction	9

PART I
1. All About Walking	17
2. Your Walking Fitness Program: Before You Start	45
3. Seven-Week Beginner Walking Fitness Program	73
4. The Ultimate Guide to Outdoor Walking	81
5. Indoor Walking: Don't Let the Weather Put You Off	112
6. Make It a Lifestyle: Creating a Habit of Walking	127
7. Tracking, Monitoring, and Measuring Your Results	136

PART II
8. High-Quality Nutrition and Healthy Foods to Support Your Walks	155
9. Tracking and Monitoring Your Weight Loss	165
Conclusion	179
References	183

INTERMITTENT FASTING FOR WOMEN
Healthfit Publishing

Introduction	203

Part I
ALL ABOUT INTERMITTENT FASTING

1. The What, Why, and How of Intermittent Fasting	211
2. Why Choose Intermittent Fasting?	228
3. Popular Types of Intermittent Fasting	240
4. Women and Fasting, Diet, and Exercise	255
5. Intermittent Fasting: How to Start	273

Part II
BONUS: EASY EXERCISES TO BOOST YOUR FASTING

6. Walking to a Slimmer, Fitter, and Healthier You	309
7. Maximize Your Walking Workout With These Tips	325
Conclusion	363
References	367
Also by Healthfit Publishing	387

WALKING YOUR WAY TO WEIGHT LOSS

A SIMPLE TWO-PART APPROACH TO
BECOMING FITTER, HEALTHIER, AND
HAPPIER IN 49 DAYS

HEALTHFIT PUBLISHING

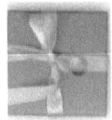 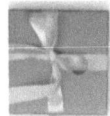

A Free Bonus To Our Readers

To get you started on your walking journey, we have created:

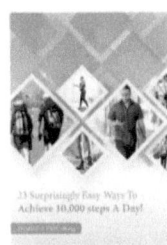 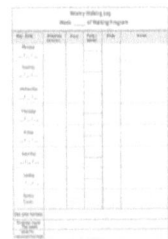 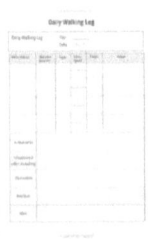 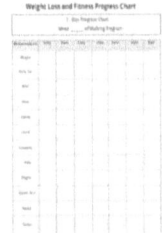

Free Bonus #1
23 Easy Ways To Achieve 10,000 Steps A Day

Free Bonus #2
A Weekly Walking Log

Free Bonus #3
A Daily Walking Log

Free Bonus #4
A Weight Loss and Fitness Progress Chart

With 23 Easy Ways to Achieve 10,000 Steps A Day, you get

- 10 health benefits of walking
- 9 risks associated with a sedentary lifestyle
- 23 different ways to achieve 10,000 steps each day

A Weekly Walking Log to record distance, time, speed/pace, steps and notes.

A Daily Walking Log to record walk/route, distance, time, pace/speed and notes.

A Weight Loss and Fitness Progress Chart to record weight, body fat, bust, hips, etc

To get your free bonuses, please click on the link or scan the QR code below and let us know the email address to send it to.

https://healthfitpublishing.com/bonus/wtwl/

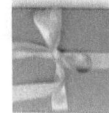 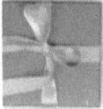

INTRODUCTION

"Walking is man's best medicine."

— HIPPOCRATES

How much time do you spend sitting around each day? It's become a way of life in a modern world dominated by sedentary professions and advancing technology that can do almost anything for us without us having to get up and do it ourselves. Where has all of this modern advancement left us and what is its legacy? It's giving us more sitting around than ever before, expanding waistlines, and a list of common medical conditions that just keeps getting longer. Aren't you

INTRODUCTION

tired of sitting, feeling less than fantastic, and battling health conditions that are sucking the joy out of your life?

If you answered 'yes,' you should be tired of it all and you have come to exactly the right place. HealthFit Publishing is dedicated to bringing you high quality, accurate, and actionable information to help you improve your life. We understand your struggles with weight loss and poor health in a world that seems to be supporting unhealthy lifestyles left, right, and center. We have the same vision and goals as you do; a happier, fitter lifestyle through the power of proper nutrition and exercise. We're here to tell you that, no matter how long you've been trying unrealistic diets and falling short of your goals, you can do this. You can achieve weight loss and health. Furthermore, you owe it to yourself. You deserve to be happy in your own skin and feel great.

You may have picked this title up and thought, "How is walking going to get me anywhere close to my dream of shedding these extra pounds?" Many people wonder that very same thing. After all, walking is gentle. How can it have the same weight loss power attributed to it as intense forms of exercise like running? That is where the humble walking workout is sorely underestimated.

Walking is one of the simplest and most effective forms of exercise. It's practically the perfect exercise. Walking is one of the very few forms of exercise available that transcends capabilities, socio-economic barriers, and even age. It doesn't matter who you are, whether you're male or female, young or old, rich, poor, in the countryside or living it large in an urban jungle, walking is accessible to virtually everybody. It can be done anywhere, at any time. All you have to do is lace up a pair of walking shoes and get moving.

Walking is more than just exercise for your body. It's an exercise for your mind and spirit as well. All it takes is as little as a 10-minute walk to give your mood a quick pick-me-up. It can also help change the way you see the world, honing your perception of smaller details and enhancing creativity. When you feel fitter, healthier, and get a dose of walking's mood-boosting, feel-good vibes, you're going to wonder why you didn't start walking ages ago.

We're going to tell you:

- What the health and weight loss benefits of walking are.
- How to set walking goals and cultivate the right mindset to achieve these goals.
- How to walk practically anywhere, from the great outdoors to more confined spaces.
- How to make the most of being indoors or working at home and sneaky tips and tricks for packing in steps toward your daily walking goal.
- What role nutrition plays in weight loss and why you should clean up your eating habits to complement your new walking program.

INTRODUCTION

- How to track everything from your fitness progress to your weight loss and why tracking is so important.
- We will also provide you with a seven-week beginner walking program with tips on how to customize it to increase the difficulty as you get fitter and start pushing yourself more.

We've all suffered setbacks in our journey toward a healthy weight and feeling great. Many of us have been duped into following fad diets and flash-in-the-pan exercise routines, and fallen prey to yo-yo dieting. It's everywhere. You can't turn a corner or look at any form of media without being bombarded by the latest celebrity fitness tricks and the newest "must try" diet that will "solve all your weight loss woes."

So, what makes walking different? Walking is tried, trusted, and has stood the test of time to prove its worth as a powerful health, fitness, and weight loss tool. For many people, it's the only tool they really use. Walking is the best decision you will ever make for your health and happiness and we're going to show you how to do it right, setting you up for success from the very first step. What are you waiting for? The life you want to live is right around the corner. Keep reading to get started and never look back.

ABOUT HEALTHFIT PUBLISHING

Healthfit Publishing is a health and wellness publishing brand. Our mission is to bring sound, actionable knowledge and advice straight from the health and wellness industry to readers from all walks of life. Our focus is on simple lifestyle changes that are easy to make for improving your overall quality of life.

We are made up of a diverse group of dynamic individuals who are passionate about inspiring and motivating others to achieve their health, fitness, and weight loss goals. Our team members are well-respected in their fields and bring expertise and experience in wellness, health, fitness, nutrition, and meticulous research to the table. We are dedicated to making healthy living accessible to anyone who is interested in transforming their life and boosting their happiness by improving their wellbeing.

Our team's diversity is our strong point and the common thread that brings us together is a zest for living life to its fullest and a passion for healthy living. Exercise and good nutrition are just two of our top interests and it's not hard to find inspiration in either.

PART I

1

ALL ABOUT WALKING

Live to walk. Walk to live. When someone mentions exercise, the image your mind conjures up probably involves high-intensity aerobics classes and running on a treadmill. This isn't actually the case. We're going to redefine how you view and interpret exercise.

The Cambridge Dictionary defines exercise as:

"physical activity that you do to make your body strong and healthy" (Cambridge Dictionary. (n.d.). Exercise)

By this definition, the activity that gets you moving to improve your physical health is exercise and that includes walking. Walking is the most basic form of exercise and it is accessible to pretty much everyone. Walking as exercise can and will help you lose weight and improve your health and

I'm going to tell you why and how to walk your way to a slimmer, healthier, and happier you.

THE PERILS OF A SEDENTARY LIFESTYLE

Before we dive into the many health benefits of walking, perhaps we should take a closer look at why a sedentary lifestyle is so bad for you. Modern life has become increasingly sedentary. More and more people's work is leaving them office-bound. Technology is one of the biggest culprits for fewer people spending time outdoors for leisure activities and entertainment. Commuting for hours a day to get to and from work often sees them sitting. Life, as we know it, is about sitting and all of this sitting is impacting health in ways you may not even realize.

The dangers of living a predominantly sedentary lifestyle include:

- Anxiety.
- Breast cancer.
- Cardiovascular disease.
- Colon cancer.
- Computer vision syndrome (eye strain caused by looking at a computer or tablet screen for extended periods of time).
- Depression.
- Diabetes.
- Gout.

- High blood pressure.
- Lipid problems.
- Lower back pain caused by herniated disks.
- Migraines.
- Mortality in adults.
- Obesity.
- Osteoporosis.
- Scoliosis.
- Skin problems including hair loss.

THE BENEFITS OF WALKING

You may not realize just how many benefits walking can offer you. Weight loss and improved physical fitness are two of the biggest and most obvious benefits, but those are not all that should motivate you to lace up a pair of walking shoes and start pounding the pavement.

Weight Loss

Walking will help you lose weight in several ways. When all of these effects come together, you will notice the pounds start melting away.

- Your metabolism will get a boost, which will lead to your body burning more calories per day than you do right now.
- Walking can help develop muscle and combat muscle loss as you get older. Muscle burns more calories

than fat. The more muscle you have, the more calories your body will naturally burn every day.
- Walking may improve how your body responds to weight loss, reducing fat around your midsection.
- Walking can mimic high-intensity interval training (HIIT) when done in alternating intervals between a faster and slower pace. The result is increased calorie burn after you have finished your walk.

Accessibility and Suitability

Walking is accessible and suitable for virtually everybody.

- It won't cost you a cent; no hefty gym membership fees required.
- You can also take a walk anywhere that is designated for pedestrians, from pavements, to walking paths, to the great outdoors.
- Walking is such a gentle form of exercise; it's suitable for anybody regardless of their age or body type.
- You don't need any equipment for walking and you can do it at any time.

Healthier Heart

Regular walking can help improve the health of your ticker, lowering your risk of developing serious heart disease and even recovering from having bypass surgery or a heart attack. Walking and following a healthy diet can reduce plaque build-up in the arteries supplying your heart with blood. It is also associated with a lower resting heart rate, meaning your heart doesn't have to work as hard at rest and while getting physical.

High blood pressure is a factor in developing heart disease. Your heart is put under increased stress when it has to work harder to pump blood. This added stress can weaken the muscle over time and cause enlargement. A weaker heart muscle puts you at risk of heart failure. Another risk associated with an enlarged heart is a higher susceptibility to forming blood clots that could get lodged in an artery and prevent vital organs from getting blood.

Plaque buildup in your coronary arteries is the root of heart disease. It narrows the arteries supplying blood to the heart, limiting the amount of oxygen it gets. When your love muscle can't get enough oxygen, it can't function properly. As if that isn't bad enough, should that plaque build-up get so bad it narrows the artery too much, a blood clot can get stuck and cut off blood flow to your heart. Your heart can also experience a lack of blood flow to it if the plaque completely blocks the artery. If either of these two scenarios happens, parts of your heart may die.

How does walking help? Walking helps make the blood vessels more flexible which allows blood to flow more easily through them, lowering your blood pressure. Walking also keeps the cells of your arteries healthier so that they can keep producing small amounts of nitrous oxide. Nitrous oxide produced by these arterial cells helps to prevent arterial blocks from occurring.

Diabetes

Taking a walk after meals is associated with lower blood sugar levels. Lowering your blood sugar levels reduces your risk of developing insulin resistance; a precursor to type 2 diabetes. Constantly having too much insulin in your blood eventually renders the insulin ineffective at removing glucose from your blood, increasing your overall blood sugar levels. Higher blood sugar levels could turn into type 2 diabetes if left untreated.

Note: Insulin resistance is discussed in further detail in Chapter 8.

TEN THOUSAND STEPS A DAY

Walking 10,000 steps a day may seem like a tall order, but you'd be surprised how easy it can be. Not only is it an achievable fitness goal, but it is also a great target for starting out your walking to weight loss journey.

Origins

In 1964, two things happened in Japan. The country was gearing up for the Tokyo Olympics and modern pedometers were introduced. Japan already had a growing awareness of increasing lifestyle-related diseases and that exercise could reduce the risk of developing those diseases. Hosting the

Olympics increased the population's fitness focus. Pedometers became readily available and helped people keep track of how many steps they took and how far they walked daily, contributing to their desire to increase their fitness.

In the Japanese language, manpo-kei translates to 10,000 steps. Those dedicated to taking more steps per day developed manpo-kei as a slogan and walking clubs started popping up in response to the increase in the number of walkers. Manpo-kei was set as the minimum daily step goal. A goal of 10,000 steps per day has since spread to walkers across the globe.

Between 2005 and 2006, the Ghent University in Belgium and the Queensland University-based School of Human Movement Studies collaborated to perform the Ghent Study. The study's objective was to determine how valid this manpo-kei concept was for increasing overall health and fitness. The participants ranged from individuals interested in improved health and fitness to those who had an increased risk of developing chronic diseases such as heart disease and type 2 diabetes. The study was successful and participants who managed to make their manpo-kei daily step goal reported an improved feeling of overall well-being.

Application

Aiming for 10,000 steps per day is a good goal for anybody who is starting to walk for fitness. However, this could seem like a daunting task and an unachievable goal to those who lead a sedentary lifestyle. You can reach this goal by taking a 30- to 60-minute dedicated walk per day, but this might be asking a bit much of someone leading a very inactive lifestyle. Don't worry, you can work your way up to that manpo-kei goal by first tracking your average daily steps using a pedometer of some kind. Once you have a good baseline to work with, begin adding 2,000 to 2,500 steps to your daily baseline and work your way up to 10,000 steps by gradually increasing the number of steps you take a day.

Diet and Intensity

Walking your way to weight loss and fitness is about more than just walking. Walking alone isn't going to do all the work when it comes to shedding the weight. It is important to realize that taking a leisurely stroll and eating an unbalanced diet isn't going to do much good. The intensity of your walking and following a healthy, calorie-controlled diet are essential factors for your walking for weight loss goal.

The speed at which you walk, the terrain you walk on, and even the style of walking all contribute to the calorie-burning ante of your walks. You don't have to start out trying to out-walk champion speed walkers. Gradually step it up to increase your pace and vary the terrain to include more challenging inclines.

While exercise is a vital component of weight loss, fitness, and overall health, it is not effective on its own. Eating a healthy, balanced diet and creating a calorie deficit is crucial to success. Increasing your daily walking goal to 10,000 steps per day is a great way to start burning off those calories to create the deficit you need to lose weight.

We'll take a more in-depth look at diet in a later chapter.

WALK TO WEIGHT LOSS WITH THE RIGHT MINDSET

When you embark on any life-changing journey, such as walking for weight loss, you must cultivate the right mindset to help you stay motivated. It's not always going to be easy. There are going to be days you're tempted to be lazy, bad weather days, and even other people who will try to get you to skip your walk in favor of other leisure activities. When you have the right mindset, you can resist the things that tempt you to cheat on your walking program under the premise of *I'll get back to it tomorrow. One day won't hurt, right?*

The problem with playing hooky on your walking goals is that it will only hurt you, not help you. It can be a slippery slope, leading to more and more days where you don't reach your goal. Before you know it, you could be right back where you started in the first place. Get your head in the game to develop a rock-solid resolve to stay motivated and reach your goals. After all, you are doing this for yourself, and it's what you really want, so don't cheat yourself out of health, fitness, and the slimmer body you're starting a walking program to achieve.

Setting Goals

Setting goals is your blueprint outlining what you want to achieve and how you're going to get there. Goals are great motivators, but you must not set them willy-nilly. Setting goals is a process that requires consideration.

Set Realistic Goals

One of the key factors to achieving your goals is setting reasonable, realistic ones. Set your goals before you even start your walking program, but be realistic. All you are doing by setting big goals from the start is setting yourself up for failure.

Start out small. As the saying goes, *"You must learn to crawl before you can learn to walk."* This is true of setting your walking goals. Set lower, more easily attainable goals in the beginning, to avoid discouraging yourself if you don't meet them according to your timeline. Reaching goals is a great motivator, but not reaching them can put you off walking altogether.

Set goals that are realistic on a personal level. The internet is chock-full of amazing before and after photos, dramatic fast weight loss stories, and peppy blog posts about making significant progress at the speed of light. It can be difficult to separate reality from what we see online, even though it's often unrealistic. Don't try to set goals according to the standards or stories of others, but set them according to what you can realistically achieve for yourself.

When setting goals for your progress toward weight loss and overall health, don't try to overload yourself with a dozen goals at once. Pick one goal and stick with it. Focusing on one goal at a time will help you measure success better. If you make progress toward that goal, you won't be discouraged if you aren't making progress toward another goal at the same time.

Important note: Tell your friends, family, and your general support system about your intention to make changes and to start walking your way to a slimmer, healthier, and happier you. Telling other people helps keep you motivated to hold yourself accountable for your efforts and it makes others hold you accountable as well.

Specific, Measurable, and Timed

When setting your goals, it's not only important to make them realistic and personally achievable. It's vital to make them:

- Specific.
- Measurable.
- Time-bound.

Be as specific as possible with each goal. One of the mistakes that people often make when setting goals is being too vague. For instance, many people set their goal as losing weight. What does this mean and how do you measure your progress and success if you don't know what your goal weight is. Set a specific weight loss goal of X number of pounds. Setting a specific weight loss goal will make your progress measurable. You can measure how far you've come and how far you have to go to reach your goal.

The final factor about being specific and measurable is to set a time limit on how long you have to reach your goal. Even if you set a specific weight loss goal, if you don't set a time by which you want to have reached that goal, you could be working toward it indefinitely. For example, if you set your weight loss goal as losing 10 pounds, if you don't set a time limit, you could become lax with your walking to weight loss program and it could take you years to reach that goal. Set a realistic timeline. Don't risk becoming discouraged because you haven't reached a realistic goal in an unrealistic time frame.

Mission Statement: Making the Commitment

A mission statement, or intention statement, is a vital part of setting goals and sticking to them. It's a summary of your goals and your commitment to meeting them. It also serves as a reminder and motivation to keep working toward your goals.

Your mission statement isn't going to detail exactly how you're going to go about achieving your goals. It's there to help you maintain focus on the days when your motivation to walk wavers due to the stresses you experience on a daily basis. You may even alter your mission statement as you make progress, reach your current goals, and set new ones.

Mission Statement Components

Writing down a goal actually has the psychological effect of solidifying your determination to make it happen. Write it out with pen and paper; don't just type it up on a computer or your phone. You can keep a digital copy on your gadgets for ease of access, but make sure you physically write it down.

Make time to read your mission statement daily. Rereading your goals and intentions is both a reminder and motivation to keep going. A mission statement won't just include your goals; it will detail your values and motivation behind your goals.

When writing your mission statement, write down a specific, measurable goal and the timeframe you want to achieve it in. Your statement could look something like this:

- Walk 10,000 steps per day.
- Eat a healthy, balanced diet.
- Control my calorie intake, X number of calories per day.

Exercise: Write Your Mission Statement

- *Write down your goals. Be specific.*

- *Write down why you want to make changes to reach those goals.* What is your motivation for starting a walking program? Also, write down what you project the outcome would be if you didn't make these changes to your lifestyle.
- *Write down some important points you want to emphasize and keep them in mind often.* They could be anything from ideas of how your life will be changed for the better to asking yourself crucial questions about why you are undertaking a walking program. Don't try to write too many points down; pick a few that you can easily remember without having to refer to your mission statement to be reminded of them.
- *Write down obstacles you think you may face along your weight loss journey.* Try to think about things that would trigger you to not reach your goals. For instance, you may anticipate that a busy day will deter you from achieving your manpo-kei goal. Come up with reasonable counter solutions to help you overcome those obstacles.
- *The last thing you are going to do is sign your mission statement.* Not only does writing it down increase your determination, but signing it makes it personal, it seals the deal, and makes you even more determined.

Stay Motivated

Staying motivated can sometimes be difficult. You could be tempted to 'cheat' on your diet or you may be feeling tired or too busy to make your daily step goal. There are many things that could affect your motivation on any given day. Here are some tips to help you keep that motivation alive so that you do continue to work toward your goals.

- Read your mission statement regularly to remind yourself of the reasons behind making this change and starting a walking program.
- Focus on the progress you are making toward your goals instead of how far you may still have to go.
- Keep a walking and weight loss journal to track your daily diet (every single meal, snack, etc.), your walking and step count per day, how you feel, and the emotions you experience. You can even write down how you overcome obstacles to reflect upon when other obstacles crop up.
- Keep your self-talk and thoughts positive. Self-talk is the inner dialogue you have about yourself. If you tell yourself that you aren't making progress, you are less likely to stay motivated to keep working toward your goal.
- Find walking groups or a walking buddy who will motivate you when you feel unmotivated and hold you accountable for your diet and walking progress. It also helps to make you feel less alone in your

efforts when you have company to share the experiences with.
- If you know of anybody who has undertaken a walking program for health and weight loss, use them as a role model. If you don't have a walking role model, find a person with a body structure similar to yours at your goal weight or size. When you have someone to look up to as having achieved the same kind of goals you have or having the body you are working toward, it can bump up your motivation on days when it's lacking. After all, if they did it, so can you.
- Work walking into your lifestyle so that you aren't trying to do something that just doesn't fit into your daily life. For instance, if you cannot take a dedicated walk every day to make your step goal, find ways to get those steps in, like parking further from the grocery store doors or taking the stairs instead of an escalator or elevator.
- Celebrate reaching your goals. You don't have to celebrate with a meal, especially if your goal is weight loss. You can treat yourself to some pampering, like a facial, or to something you've wanted, like that dress you've been eyeing in the store.
- If you don't make the progress you expect, don't get discouraged. Yes, you want to shed some extra weight, but it will also do wonders for your overall

health. Ultimately, any weight you lose is good for your health and you are making an effort toward overall improvement. Every little bit of progress you make should be seen and celebrated as a win.
- Get a dog. Yes, really. A dog is not only a fantastic companion, but you will be responsible for walking your dog every day. This is a responsibility you can't get out of just because you don't feel like walking. A furry friend will also make walking less lonely and keep you motivated to get up and make your step goal.
- Find spaces to walk in that you enjoy, even if you can only make it to them once or twice a week. The idea is to make it as much fun as possible as often as possible. You are more likely to stay motivated if you enjoy your walks.

COMMON WALKING CONCERNS AND SOLUTIONS

Walking is simple and easy, but it's not without its potential concerns. Don't let common concerns such as shoddy knees or weather deter you from your walking plan, as we have the solutions for you right here.

What if the Weather Is Cold or Hot?

When you take dedicated walks outdoors, the weather can be of concern. Nobody wants to get hypothermia or heat stroke, so how do you get around the weather?

- Layer up when it's cold outside.
- When it's hot, try walking in the cooler early and later hours of the day. Alternatively, try going for a few short walks throughout the day.
- If the weather is really terrible, try walking indoors or using equipment such as a treadmill.

How Much Water Is Enough?

Staying hydrated is a very important part of taking a walk, especially if you're going for a longer walk. Your hydration needs are as individual as you are and depend on various factors such as your weight, the temperature and humidity levels, and your individual perspiration rate. Due to the personal nature of your hydration needs, there is no cut and dried answer.

Weigh yourself before going for a walk and again when you get back. If you haven't had any water to drink along the way, you should have lost weight. Each pound lighter you are suggests that you should drink 16 ounces of water to compensate. For instance, if you lost two pounds during your walk, you will need to drink 32 ounces of water.

Sports drinks are a good idea for longer walks of an hour or more. These drinks contain electrolytes to replenish the ones you are sweating out.

What About Boredom?

If you find that you are getting bored of the same old route day in and day out, try taking a different route, walking in a different area, or switching up the terrain. If changing to a different route isn't an option, try joining a walking club or buddying up with a friend to keep you company. If neither of those options works for you, keep your mind busy during your walk by listening to an audiobook or podcast.

Important note: If you are listening to music, a podcast, an audiobook, or anything else during your walk, always make sure you can hear what is going on around you. Be careful not to get so absorbed in what you are listening to that you lose touch with your surroundings. It can become dangerous if you are unaware of what is happening around you.

What if There Isn't Enough Time?

There is always time for a walk, even if it's only 10 minutes. It can be difficult to make your step goal on days when you're short on time, but that doesn't mean you have to give up on your walking program altogether for the day. A 10-minute walk is better than no walk at all.

If you're out of time to fit a full-length walk into your day, make those 10 minutes count by increasing the difficulty to bump up your calorie burn by considering these techniques:

- Make use of inclines.

- Vary your pace at intervals to get a HIIT walking workout in.
- Add some basic bodyweight exercises to your walks such as step-ups, lunges, and squats.

Do Your Knees Hurt?

Knee pain can occur either during or after a walk. Your first port of call to treat and prevent knee pain should be your footwear. Wearing the correct shoes that fit properly and aren't worn is important to prevent a variety of uncomfortable or even painful niggles such as sore knees. Follow these tips as well:

- Make sure your stride is correct and that you are not taking steps that are too big or overstriding.
- Don't push your weekly walking distance up by more than 10% week-to-week to prevent pushing your body too hard, too quickly.
- Ice painful body areas after your walk to decrease any inflammation.
- Stretch after your walk to increase your flexibility.

Important note: If your knee pain is extreme or the problem continues despite your efforts, it's time to see a medical professional.

Can Side Stitches Be Prevented or Stopped?

What are side stitches really and what causes them? When you get a stitch in your side, it's because your diaphragm is in spasm. Side stitches often happen when you are breathing hard or fast. To avoid side stitches:

- Allow your body to warm up properly at the beginning of your walk before stepping up the pace later on. This may help prevent a side stitch from starting.
- If you experience a side stitch that becomes very painful, slow down or even stop for a short while until the pain subsides.
- Avoid eating or drinking too much shortly before you go for a walk to help prevent side stitches.

What if You're Sore After a Walk?

Sore and stiff muscles are a normal part of post-workout life. Even walking can result in post-walk soreness, especially if you're a newcomer to the world of walking for weight loss and fitness. The initial soreness should ease up as you get into the swing of things and shouldn't last more than a day or two or prevent you from going on your next dedicated walk. To limit the soreness and stiffness, always:

- Stretch out properly.
- Ice sore spots after your walk.

- Take a break from walking for a day or two until the soreness goes away.
- Take a short and easy recovery walk the day after a long, strenuous walk to get the muscles moving and blood flowing without putting too much pressure on your already sore body.

Can You Overtrain While Walking?

The answer is yes, you can overtrain while walking. Walking is like any other endurance exercise; you want to increase your distance, but not too quickly. Putting in too much mileage or upping the pace too quickly can lead to overtraining and injury. Take note of the following concepts:

- Prevent overtraining by only increasing your effort (either mileage or speed) by approximately 10% per week.
- Increase your recovery time between walks if you are still stiff and sore from your last walk by the time you need to go for your next one.

What About Lacking Energy?

If you get halfway through a walk and don't feel like you have the energy to finish it, you may want to rethink your pre-walk nutrition. If you're eating before a walk, what are you eating? If you're not eating before a walk, how do you expect your body to have fuel to burn while you're walking?

Here are some ideas to provide adequate fuel for your walks:

- Eat simple carbohydrates that are easy to digest for quick energy release.
- If your walk is going to be 30 minutes or less, a piece of toast or a banana should keep you going.
- If you are going to be walking for more than an hour or will be increasing the intensity of your walk, consider something with a little more oomph like a smoothie or a small portion of oatmeal.

Tip: Find your ideal pre-walk nutrition by experimenting with different foods and keeping track of how what you eat makes you feel during and after your walk.

FOOTWEAR FOR SUCCESS

Walking shoes are called walking shoes for a reason. They have been designed specifically for that exact purpose. Their unique features make walking as efficient and comfortable as possible and you shouldn't start a walking program without having the correct walking shoes first.

Wearing proper walking shoes that fit well will not only make your walk more comfortable, but they can also actually prevent you from suffering injuries that may put you off walking. Some of the injuries good shoes can help prevent include knee pain, calluses, and painful blisters. So, how do you go about choosing the perfect shoe to get you started and keep you walking?

Basic Parts of a Walking Shoe

Before you can even start shopping for and trying on walking shoes, you need to know what the basic parts of the shoes are. Knowing which parts are which and what they do will help you look for and recognize a perfect fit:

- *Achilles tendon protector:* The very back upper part of the shoe that rests against your Achilles tendon and holds the shoe around your heel to reduce stress on your Achilles tendon.
- *Heel collar:* The upper part of the shoe that fits around your ankle, cushioning it and holding the shoe in place.
- *Toe box:* The upper front part of the shoe where your toes go should be spacious enough to prevent blisters and calluses.
- *Toe cap:* The very front part of the shoe upper around the front of your toes.
- *Upper:* The upper front part of the shoe that holds your foot in the shoe. Common materials for an upper include synthetic material, mesh, and leather. When looking for a walking shoe, consider a mesh upper for a lightweight and breathable shoe.
- *Insole:* The top layer of the bottom of the shoe that your foot comes in contact with. It supports the arch

of your food and offers cushioning. Some insoles are made to be removable so they can be cleaned of sweat and dirt.
- *Midsole:* The layer of the bottom of the shoe between the outsole and the insole. It further supports and cushions your foot to decrease the impact of your foot hitting the ground. Common midsole materials include air, foam, and gel.
- *Outsole:* The bottom layer of the sole that comes in contact with the ground. The tread and grooves of the outsole offer grip.

Foot Shape

Foot shape is something you should consider when shopping for a pair of walking shoes. The shoe should fit your foot; your foot shouldn't be forced to fit the shoe. Comfortable walking shoes are crucial to your enjoyment of walking and sticking with your walking program. After all, who's going to want to walk if their feet hurt?

Length and Width

How wide and long are your feet? Shoes come in a variety of shapes and sizes, just like feet. Ensure that your shoes fit snugly. Too wide, too narrow, or not enough toe room and you could end up with blisters, calluses, hammertoes, or bunions; all of which are painful.

Arches

Your foot arches help your feet to adapt to different surfaces and distribute your weight evenly across your feet. They are made up of bones, muscles, tendons, and ligaments that move. While arches may vary slightly from person to person, there are three main types of arches:

High arches: High-arched feet may not absorb impact well, potentially contributing to strain placed on your joints and muscles. Shoes with cushioning for shock absorption and a curved sole shape are the most suitable.

Low arches: Low-arched feet are commonly referred to as flat feet. Choose a walking shoe with motion control for stability and a straighter sole shape.

Neutral arches: As the name implies, neutral arches are neither significantly flat nor too arched. Opt for a shoe with a straighter or semi-curved sole shape and firm midsole, and some stability at the back of the foot.

Fit Tips

Your feet swell during the day. The best time of day for shoe shopping is later in the day when they have swollen up a bit. Shoe shopping first thing in the morning could fool you into buying shoes that will be uncomfortably tight for afternoon walks.

- Try walking shoes on wearing the same socks you will wear for walking.
- Shop at a store that has a variety of styles. Try on different brands and types of shoes to find your perfect fit.
- Don't just buy the same size and arch shape you have always bought. Your foot shape can and may actually change over time.
- It's normal to have one foot that is bigger than the other. Try on shoes in a size that fits your bigger foot.
- Don't try to convince yourself that a shoe will mold itself to your foot after a few walks. Shoes should be completely comfortable to walk in from the moment you first put them on. Don't just try on one shoe and buy the pair. Try on both shoes, wiggle your toes around, and take a walk around the store to test them out.
- The shoe should fit snugly, not tightly.
- Ladies with wide feet shouldn't be shy to try on men's shoes. Men's shoes are typically cut bigger and could be more comfortable.
- Toe room is important. If you can't wiggle your toes or the tip of your longest toe isn't finger-width from the front of the shoe, try on a bigger size.

A Word on Worn-Out Shoes

Every shoe has a *best before* timeframe, unless you never wear them. As you walk, your shoes will incur wear and tear. You should replace your shoes regularly, even if they still look and feel fine. There could be wear that isn't visible to you, but could affect your walking comfort over time, such as a loss of support or not absorbing impact shock as well anymore.

When should you replace your walking shoes?

- After 300 to 400 miles walked in them.
- The outsole is showing obvious signs of wear.
- They aren't as comfortable as they used to be.

TAKING THE NEXT STEP

So, now you know why walking is such a great form of exercise for health and weight loss, you've set your goals, and you've picked out the perfect pair of walking shoes. It's time to take the next step in your walking for weight loss journey. It's also time to get started with a good walking fitness program to start shedding those pounds.

2

YOUR WALKING FITNESS PROGRAM: BEFORE YOU START

Deciding to get up and start walking for fitness and weight loss is the first step in the right direction, but that doesn't mean you should just slip on a pair of walking shoes and hit the streets. You need to have a game plan in place. You need to build your walking program, tailor it to accommodate your personal fitness level and abilities, and to meet your own goals.

BEFORE YOU START

Before you can start a walking fitness program, there are a few things you need to take into account to ensure that you are getting the most out of walking.

Consult a Doctor

Consult your family doctor about starting a walking program. This is especially important if you:

- Are pregnant.
- Have high blood pressure.
- Are a diabetic.
- Have a diagnosed heart condition.
- Experience chest pain, either with or without physical exertion.
- Are older than 65 years and not doing any form of exercise right now.
- Frequently experience faintness or dizziness.
- Have been leading a sedentary lifestyle for 12 months or more.
- Have any other medical condition or concern not mentioned.

Important note: It is always recommended to consult a medical practitioner before you make any lifestyle changes that may impact your health. Only a trained medical professional can give you the all-clear and provide advice based on your medical history and current health.

Get the Right Gear

Invest in basic walking gear such as shoes and clothing. You don't have to fork out for expensive fashion-forward brands, but you should invest in quality shoes and clothing. What you walk in will make a difference to how enjoyable your walking is.

- Wear loose, lightweight clothing that fits comfortably. Heavy fabrics may chafe.
- Your base layer should be made of a sweat-wicking fabric irrespective of hot or cold weather.
- Layer up in light layers that can be taken off if the temperature rises during your walk.
- Choose athletic socks over cotton socks to help prevent blisters.
- Pay special attention to your shoes. Please refer to Chapter 1 for a guide to picking out the right walking shoes.

Walking Technique

It may seem silly. You've been walking all your life since you took your first step as a toddler, right? You walk every day. Yes, you can walk but are you walking properly? Pay attention to your posture when you walk. Are you using your arms? Are you walking with the correct technique to prevent injury? Walking is a safe form of exercise, but you can still injure yourself if you aren't walking with the proper technique.

- Keep your head up with your chin in a neutral position. Don't look down or hold your head up too high.

- Lengthen your spine. Don't slouch.
- Shoulders back and down. Don't lift or round your shoulders.
- Keep your elbows slightly bent and swing your arms gently from the shoulder. Don't swing them across your body or up too high. Swing your arms at midsection height, not chest height. Swinging your arms during walking helps turn a walk into a full-body workout and can increase your calorie burn by between 5 and 10 percent.
- Keep your hips level while walking. Don't roll your hips.
- Steps should be taken from heel to toe, placing your heel down first in a rolling motion toward your toes to push off the ground again.
- Keep stride length comfortable. Don't overstride.
- Determine your ideal stride length by standing with your feet shoulder-width apart. Shift your weight forward and lean forward from your ankles. When you feel as though you are about to fall forward, put your foot out only as much as you need to prevent falling. The distance between your feet is your ideal stride length regardless of the type and pace of walking.
- Always maintain one foot on the ground at all times.
- Try not to slap your feet against the ground; it should be a controlled, smooth movement throughout your walk.

- Avoid taking longer strides, but rather take quicker steps to increase your speed.

WARM UP, COOL DOWN, AND STRETCH

Warming up, cooling down, and stretching are important aspects of walking for fitness and they are often overlooked. Perhaps it's because people don't see warming up and stretching as exercise. Perhaps they don't understand just how much warming up and stretching can actually benefit them. Whatever the reason for others overlooking a good warm-up and stretch, you shouldn't, and here's why:

- Warming up gets your body moving and increases your body temperature. Your muscles will thank you for warming up because they get more oxygen as they get warmer. In turn, your muscles can move better, contract, and relax more easily, preventing muscle strain. As a muscle, your heart also warms up for action which prevents unnecessary strain during your walk.
- When your muscles are warmed up and more elastic, your risk of injury decreases. If you've ever pulled or strained a muscle, you'll know how painful it can be and how long it takes to heal properly. Pulling or straining a leg muscle on a walk is no fun, especially when you consider that you have to use that muscle

to get back home again, which could cause further injury.
- Warming up and stretching your muscles further prevents injury by increasing your flexibility and range of motion. The more flexible you are and the better your range of motion, the less restricted your movement and the less chance there is of suffering injury if you do happen to stumble.

Important note: In times gone by, people may have stretched before getting their muscles warmed up. Don't make that mistake. Always stretch after your warm-up. Getting your muscles warm and elastic or stretchy will improve the efficacy of stretching and prevent injury from trying to stretch out cold, stiff muscles.

How to Warm Up

Warm up before you stretch it all out. A simple warm-up of marching in place or walking at a slow pace will do the trick. You just want to get your body moving and your muscles warmed up. You don't want to put your body through its paces just yet. Warming up shouldn't take too long—only a few minutes—but we'll give you a better idea of how long to warm up when we get to your walking program.

Stretches for Walking

Feet: Without your feet, you can't walk. Your feet are jam-packed with muscles, tendons, ligaments, and joints. Warming and stretching your feet before a walk can increase the range of motion and flexibility in your ankles, preventing injuries like sprains.

Calves: These powerful muscles at the back of your lower legs do a lot of work while you're walking, stretching, and contracting with each step. Stretching your calf muscles helps to prevent cramping during and after your walk.

Quadriceps: Your quads are the large muscles on the fronts of your thighs. These powerhouses support your stability and even your stamina on long walks. Stretching helps prevent strains and cramps.

Hamstrings: Your hamstrings are the large muscles at the backs of your thighs, leading up toward your glutes. You can really feel them working if you are walking uphill. You don't want these muscles to seize up, cramp, or strain during or after your walk.

Hips: In particular, your hip flexors. These muscles run through your hips and allow you to pick your legs up when taking a step. Stretching helps lengthen them so that your range of motion while walking is better for a more comfortable walk.

The Basic Stretches

Hold each of the below stretches for 10 to 20 seconds with the exception of the ankle rotation which can be done in fluid motions. You should feel a light tension or stretching; don't force the stretch further than is comfortable to prevent injury.

If you need some extra stability while performing the stretches, hold onto a solid object. You can use pretty much anything that won't fall over if you wobble; a wall, lamp post, fence post, whatever is close by will do the job.

Ankle Rotation

You can perform an ankle rotation while sitting or standing.

- Flex your right foot, pointing your toes to feel a contraction under your foot and a stretch across the top.
- Flex your foot to bring your toes up toward you. This will stretch the underside of your foot and contract the top.
- Flex your foot to the left and right, stretching both sides of your right ankle.
- Slowly rotate your right ankle in a circle, clockwise and counterclockwise.
- Repeat the exercise with your left foot.

Calf Stretch

You can perform this stretch with or without the support of a wall or chair.

- Stand with your feet shoulder-width apart.
- Step forward with your right leg and bend the knee slightly.
- Keep your left (back) leg straight with your heel firmly planted on the ground.
- Lean forward so that you feel the stretch down the back of your calf muscle.
- Repeat with the left leg.

Hamstring Stretch

You can perform this hamstring stretch while sitting on the ground or standing up.

Sitting on the ground:

- Sit with your legs together and stretched out in front of you.
- Flex both feet upward, bringing your toes toward you, pointing up.
- Lean forward from your hips, stretching your arms out in front of you toward your toes to touch them.
- Only lean as far forward as is comfortable. If you can't touch your toes, don't force yourself.

- You should feel this stretch down the back of your thighs.

Standing:

- Stand up straight with your feet together and flat on the floor.
- Slowly bend forward from the hips, stretching your arms out toward your toes.
- Bend over as far as is comfortable for you.

Resistance Band Hamstring Stretch

- Sit with your legs together and stretched out in front of you.
- Flex both feet upward, bringing your toes toward you, pointing up.
- Loop a resistance band, towel, or rump rope around the bottom or arch of your right foot.
- Holding onto both ends, lie back on the ground.
- Bend your left knee, but keep your left foot flat on the ground.
- Raise your right leg up until it's at a 90-degree angle to the ground.
- If you can't make it all the way to a 90-degree angle, only go as far as is comfortable while still feeling the stretch down the back of your thigh.

- Keep the stretching leg as straight as possible, but don't lock your knee.
- Repeat with your left leg.

Quad Stretch

You can use a wall or chair to help you maintain your balance during this stretch.

- Stand up straight with your feet shoulder-width apart.
- Bend your right knee, bringing your right foot up toward the back of your right thigh.
- Reach around with your right hand to grab hold of your right ankle and bring it further up toward your bottom.
- Your bent right knee should be pointing straight down toward the ground.
- Don't forget to tuck your tailbone in and feel the stretch along the front of your thigh.
- Repeat with the left leg.

Groin Stretch

You might want to have a chair handy for balance support during this stretch.

- Stand with your feet wider than shoulder-width apart, but not too wide.

- Keep your right foot pointing straight ahead.
- Turn your left foot so that your toes are pointing out at a 45-degree angle.
- Keeping your right foot facing forward, lunge in the direction of your right foot.
- Don't lunge too far; only go as far as you can or until your knee is over your toes, but not past them.
- Repeat with the right leg.

Leg Swings

- Stand up straight with your feet shoulder-width apart.
- Lift your right foot off the ground and move your leg forward, tapping your toe on the ground.
- Move your leg out to the side, tapping your toes on the floor.
- Move your leg back, tapping your toes on the floor.
- Repeat with the left leg.

Hip Stretch

- Stand up straight with your feet shoulder-width apart.
- Raise your left foot off the ground, bend the knee, and bring your left foot up to cross the ankle over your right thigh.
- Slowly squat down as if you are about to sit down.

- Sit into the stretch with your right leg bent.
- Place a hand on your bent left knee and gently push down.
- You should feel the stretch in your hips.
- Repeat with the other leg.

Tip: If you can't manage to balance, even when using a chair or other support, perform this stretch while sitting on a chair or bench.

Shoulder Stretch

It's not only your legs that are working while you're walking. You are swinging your arms, and giving your shoulders a workout as well.

- Stand up straight with your feet shoulder-width apart.
- Roll your shoulders back and down.
- Raise your left arm and bring it across your chest.
- Bend your right arm at the elbow and use your right hand to gently push or pull your left arm into your chest toward your right shoulder.
- Repeat with the right arm.

The Importance of Cooling Down

So, you've warmed up, had a good walk, and now you're ready to relax, but you're not quite done yet. Before you can put your feet up and relax, you need to cool down with another round of stretching. We know that warming up helps to prevent injury, but what's so special about cooling down that you can't overlook it?

Cooling down helps prevent a sudden drop in blood pressure after a walk. Yes, walking raises your blood pressure, especially if you're walking at a fast pace and high intensity. You will also notice that your hands and feet start to swell a bit during your walk. Cooling down properly after a walk is like gradually bringing your body down from a high. It helps to stabilize your heart rate and blood pressure without allowing them to drop too quickly. It also prevents blood pooling in your lower arms and legs when your blood pressure drops as your heart rate slows down.

Cooling down stretches will help prevent what is known as DOMS or delayed onset muscle soreness. Walking is exercise and can cause muscle stiffness and soreness, especially in the beginning. It's a natural part of being physically active, but too much stiffness and soreness can hold you back from following your walking fitness program. Cool down stretches after your walk help remove lactic acid build-up in your muscles and prevent post-walk soreness.

WALKING FITNESS PROGRAM: BASIC GUIDELINES

We'll provide you with a full and clear beginner seven-week walking fitness program later in the chapter. It will provide a complete beginner walking plan with a detailed blueprint of how to get started on your walking for weight loss journey. Before we get to that, let's take a look at some simple guidelines and variables that will help you build your own walking program that can be customized to suit your personal needs. You can also use these guidelines to alter and tailor the beginner program as you progress.

Beginner Guidelines

- Walk at a brisk pace of 3 to 3.5 miles per hour. Walking a mile should take approximately 17 to 20 minutes.
- For the first three weeks, start out walking 10 minutes per day.
- After three weeks, bump up your walking time by five minutes each week until you can take a 30-minute walk six days per week.

Intermediate Guidelines

- Walk at a pace of 3.5 to 4.5 miles per hour. Walking a mile should take approximately 13 to 17 minutes.
- Take a 3-mile walk three to five times a week. A 3-mile walk should take around 45 minutes.
- If you can't manage a pace of 3.5 to 4.5 miles per hour, slow the pace down and extend the distance/walking time.

Advanced Guidelines

- If you can comfortably manage walking according to the intermediate guidelines above, it may be time to switch things up a bit and take your walking to the next level.
- Take your walk to the beach, if you live on the coast. The soft, loose sand will increase the resistance of your walk, making it more challenging.
- Add inclines to increase intensity.
- Go off road by taking a hike in a scenic area with variable terrain for increasing intensity on different sections of your walk.
- If your regular walking route takes you past staircases, start climbing those stairs as part of your walking program.
- Add some light handheld or wrist weights and keep swinging those arms to increase the amount of effort you exert. Start off with lighter weights of around two to three pounds.
- You could give racewalking a try. Racewalking is fast-paced at five to nine miles per hour and you may be surprised to discover that there are local groups, organizations, and even competitions in your area.
- Give rucking a try.

What is Rucking?

Rucking is the term for a popular way to up your walking ante based on an age-old military practice. The military has been practicing rucking for centuries from the Spartans to the Romans to modern-day soldiers. Rucking is considered to be the foundation upon which Special Forces training is based. It is the practice of carrying a rucksack, or backpack, loaded with supplies and provisions for miles or even days at a time.

Modern walkers have adopted the concept to bump up the intensity of their walking workout. Rucking has become a fun and effective variation that takes traditional walking to a whole new level.

- Get a rucksack or backpack. Invest in a good quality bag that fits comfortably and distributes weight evenly across your shoulders and back. Thickly padded shoulder straps offer added comfort, especially if you're loading the rucksack up with heavier weight.
- Add a challenging, but comfortable, amount of weight to the bag. You don't want to make the weight too heavy when you start out. You can gradually increase the weight as you get stronger and fitter. A good starting point is to use 10 percent of your body weight and gradually increase it.

- You can use just about anything to weigh down your rucksack, but it should be comfortable, not oddly shaped, and not poke, bump, or chafe while walking. Some ideas include sandbags, one-gallon water bottles, and specialized rucking weight plates.
- Ensure that the weight is evenly distributed and stable close to your back. The rucksack should sit high against your back, not sag low against your lower back.
- Strap on your weighted rucksack and start walking. When you start rucking, try to aim for a 30-minute walk and build yourself up to walking for an hour or more at a time.

Benefits of Rucking

- Improves heart health because it elevates your heart rate more than traditional walking does.
- More effort exerted means more calories burned.
- Rucking is less stressful and lower impact than running, but offers similar benefits in terms of fitness and weight loss.
- The practice of carrying a weighted bag on your back could help improve poor posture caused by spending hours in front of a computer. When done right, the force exerted on your shoulders helps to pull them back into alignment for better posture.

- Carrying a loaded rucksack while walking helps tone and shape muscles while building strength.

Strength Training

When you have worked up your walking fitness, adding strength training can help tone and increase lean muscle mass for improved fitness and help keep the pounds off.

Lower Body

While walking, your lower body is the target of the workout. Some types of walking, like Nordic walking, will throw in a bit of an upper-body workout, but the bulk of the work is being done from the waist down. You can tone and improve muscle in your lower body by adding some basic strength training to your walking workout which would create a HIIT effect. Your workout would alternate between the cardiovascular workout of walking and strength training.

Here are some suggestions for adding strength training to your walking workout:

Squats

Walk a certain distance, such as a city block, stop and perform 10 squats. Repeat this pattern three or more times during your walk. You can increase the number of times you stop to do squats as your leg strength increases.

Walking Lunges

Determine a certain distance, such as a city block. Walk for that distance and then perform walking lunges for the same distance before switching back to walking. Repeat the pattern three or more times during your walk. You can increase the number of walking lunge intervals as your leg strength increases.

For example:

- Walk a block.
- Perform lunges for a block.
- Walk a block.
- Perform lunges for a block.

It is vital that you use the correct form when performing lunges, not only to get the maximum benefit, but also to prevent injury.

- Stand with your feet shoulder-width apart.
- Step forward with your right leg.
- Bend your right knee until the knee is over your right ankle, but not past your toes.
- Bend your left knee and lower it toward the ground.
- Maintain a straight back throughout.
- Press down through your right heel to return to a standing position. Avoid pushing off with your left foot.

- Step forward with your left leg and repeat the process.

Important note: Lunges can be challenging. It is important to perform walking lunges only over a distance that is comfortable for you. You don't have to cover a whole city block. If you can only do two or three walking lunges to begin with, that's fine. You can work your way up to longer distances as you get stronger.

Modifications

If you are walking indoors, instead of using distance to indicate your strength training intervals, use a timer. Time yourself for a set period of time, such as five minutes. Alternate walking with lunges and squats at five-minute intervals.

If you cannot perform full squats and lunges, go halfway down, or as far as is comfortable for you. You can work your way up to full lunges and squats as you build leg strength.

Upper Body

Walking targets your lower body and cardiovascular system. Bring some upper body strength training into the mix for a total body workout. The best part is that you don't need heavy or bulky weights to perform the following exercises. They are all calisthenic exercises that use your body weight and can be performed virtually anywhere.

Shoulder-Blade Squeezes

- Stand with your feet shoulder-width apart.
- Raise your arms to shoulder height and bend your elbows to 90 degrees, fingers pointing toward the sky. This is called the goal-post position.
- Pull your elbows back by squeezing your shoulder blades together. It may help to imagine squeezing a stress ball between your shoulder blades.
- Release the squeeze and bring your elbows back into position.

Perform shoulder-blade squeezes for a determined distance, such as a city block, and repeat the pattern three or more times during your walk. If you are walking indoors, perform the shoulder-blade squeezes for 30 seconds at a time at set time intervals during your walk.

Lat Pull-Down

- Stand with your feet shoulder-width apart.
- Extend your arms up and outward at an angle from your sides. It may help to imagine that you are using a wide grip to hold onto a bar.
- Bend your elbows and pull your arms down until your upper arms are parallel to the ground and are roughly at shoulder height. You should feel your shoulder blades squeezing together. Imagine pulling that bar down until it is in front of your face.

- Relax your shoulders and return your arms to the starting position.

Perform lat pull-downs for a determined distance, such as a city block, and repeat the pattern three or more times during your walk. If you are walking indoors, perform the lat pull-downs for 30 seconds at a time at set time intervals during your walk.

TAILORING YOUR WALKING PROGRAM

There are three things that you can change when tailoring your walking fitness program to make it either easier or harder:

- Intensity.
- Frequency.
- Time.

Intensity

Intensity is how much effort you are putting into your walking. There are three ways to measure the intensity of your walking:

1. Talk test.
2. RPE scale self-measurement of your exertion.
3. Heart rate.

Talk Test

You can determine how much effort you are putting into your walk by talking out loud while walking.

- Easy, leisurely, or lifestyle walking: You can hold a conversation even if it's a bit breathy.
- Fitness walking: You can only have bits and pieces of a more breathless conversation while talking.
- When taking a high-intensity walk, you shouldn't be able to hold a conversation during your peak-intensity intervals.

RPE

RPE means the rate of perceived exertion. This measurement of how much effort you are putting into your workout uses a scale of 1 to 10. Unlike using a heart rate monitor, RPE is measured according to your own personal judgment of how hard you think you are exerting yourself. You can use a combination of aspects to rate your perceived exertion as accurately as possible. These aspects include:

- How fatigued you feel.
- Your heart rate.
- Your rate of breathing.
- How much you are sweating.

A rating of 1 means that your walk is super easy and a rating of 10 means that you are giving it maximum effort.

- Easy, leisurely, or lifestyle walking: You should be rating your effort between 4 and 6.
- Fitness walking: You should be rating your effort between 6 and 8.
- High-intensity walking: You should be rating your effort between 8 and 9.5.

Heart Rate

Your heart rate is directly linked to how much you are exerting yourself. Using your heart rate to determine how hard your body is working is the most accurate way to tell how much effort you are putting in. Determine your maximum heart rate:

220 − your age = your maximum heart rate (For example, if you are 30 years old, 220 - 30 = 190 beats per minute is your maximum heart rate.)

Ideal heart rates for different types of walking:

- Easy, leisurely, or lifestyle walking: 50 to 60 percent of your max heart rate.
- Fitness walking: 60 to 75 percent of your max heart rate.
- High-intensity walking: 75 to 95 percent of your max heart rate.

Tip: Don't focus on a specific heart rate, but aim for a walk that pushes your heart rate up and down across the entire ideal range for the amount of effort you want to be putting in. For example, if your maximum heart rate is 200 beats per minute and you go for a fitness walk; you should try to keep your heart rate between 120 and 150 beats per minute (60 – 75 percent).

Important note: Consult your doctor about your maximum heart rate and what your target heart rate range while walking should be if you have a heart condition, are pregnant, or take any form of medication.

Frequency

How often you walk for fitness will depend on what your goals are and how quickly you achieve them. The minimum number of times per week you should be getting your heart rate up, according to the American College of Sports Medicine, is three times weekly. If you want to lose weight through walking, you should increase that number.

A factor that influences how often you walk is the intensity of your walk. If you prefer to walk at a lower intensity, you should be walking more often. If you prefer to walk at a higher intensity, you can cut back on the number of walks you take per week. In fact, if you are walking at a very high intensity for every walk, you should be taking at least one or two days a week off to prevent overtraining, injury, and fatigue.

Time

How long your walks are depends on both the intensity and the frequency of your walks as well as a few other factors.

Intensity: High-intensity walks are likely to be shorter while low-intensity walks will be longer.

Frequency: How many times a week you choose to walk based on how intense those walks are.

Fitness level: The higher your fitness level, the longer you can sustain both low-intensity and high-intensity walks.

Personal Schedule: How much time you can dedicate to walking every day comes down to your lifestyle and schedule. You may have the time to dedicate to long walking sessions at a lower intensity. You may only have enough time to dedicate to a shorter walk at a higher intensity to meet the same goals. You can always break your walk up into several short sessions during the day if you don't have enough time to dedicate to a single walk.

Goals: How much of your available time you dedicate to walking will be influenced by your goals. If you are training toward a weight loss or walking event goal, you are probably going to spend more of your free time walking than if you are walking to maintain health and a stable weight.

THE IMPORTANCE OF TAILORING YOUR PROGRAM

Every person is different. What one person can do comfortably may be a tall order for another person. We're about to provide you with a general seven-week beginner walking program to use as a guideline. It is important to take everything you now know from this chapter and apply that knowledge to tweaking the beginner plan so that it suits your current level of fitness and your personal goals. If you are fitter or not quite fit enough, you can adjust the variables to make the plan your own.

3

SEVEN-WEEK BEGINNER WALKING FITNESS PROGRAM

To get started walking your way to a slimmer you, here's a seven-week program that you can use as-is or as a starting point to build your own program. The program starts off with walking sessions of 10 minutes (or less) and aims to increase that to 30 minutes over the first three weeks.

The days of the week are divided as follows:

- Main walking workout days are Monday, Wednesday, and Thursday.
- Walking on Tuesdays and weekends is optional to start.
- Fridays are for rest or alternative activities.

- The suggested days are only a guideline. You can arrange your walking program to suit your personal schedule.

WEEK ONE

Try for a walking pace of 3 to 3.5 miles per hour. Slow it down to 2.7 to 3 miles per hour if you can't manage that pace.

Monday	Tuesday	Wednesday	Thursday	Friday	Weekends
Warm up: 1 minute	Warm up: 1 minute	Warm up: 1 minute	Warm up: 1 minute	Rest	Warm up: 1 minute
Stretch: 2 minutes	Stretch: 2 minutes	Stretch: 2 minutes	Stretch: 2 minutes		Stretch: 2 minutes
Easy walk: 10 minutes	Easy walk: 10 minutes	Easy walk: 10 minutes	Easy walk: 10 minutes		Easy walk: 10 minutes
Stretch: 2 minutes	Stretch: 2 minutes	Stretch: 2 minutes	Stretch: 2 minutes		Stretch: 2 minutes

Remember, walking on Tuesdays and over weekends is optional to start with, as you get used to your new walking program.

WEEK TWO

Try for a walking pace of 3 to 3.5 miles per hour. Slow it down to 2.7 to 3 miles per hour if you can't manage that pace.

Monday	Tuesday	Wednesday	Thursday	Friday	Weekends
Warm up: 1 minute	Warm up: 1 minute	Warm up: 1 minute	Warm up: 1 minute	Rest	Warm up: 1 minute
Stretch: 2 minutes	Stretch: 2 minutes	Stretch: 2 minutes	Stretch: 2 minutes		Stretch: 2 minutes
Easy walk: 10 minutes	Easy walk: 10 minutes	Easy walk: 10 minutes	Easy walk: 10 minutes		Easy walk: 10 minutes
Stretch: 2 minutes	Stretch: 2 minutes	Stretch: 2 minutes	Stretch: 2 minutes		Stretch: 2 minutes

Remember, walking on Tuesdays and over weekends is optional to start with, as you get used to your new walking program.

WEEK THREE

Try for a walking pace of 3 to 3.5 miles per hour.

Monday	Tuesday	Wednesday	Thursday	Friday	Weekends
Warm up: 1 minute	Warm up: 1 minute	Warm up: 1 minute	Warm up: 1 minute	Rest	Warm up: 1 minute
Stretch: 2 minutes	Stretch: 2 minutes	Stretch: 2 minutes	Stretch: 2 minutes		Stretch: 2 minutes
Easy walk: 5 minutes	Easy walk: 10 minutes	Easy walk: 5 minutes	Easy walk: 5 minutes		Easy walk: 10 minutes
Brisk walk: 5 minutes	Stretch: 2 minutes	Brisk walk: 5 minutes	Brisk walk: 5 minutes		Stretch: 2 minutes
Stretch: 2 minutes		Stretch: 2 minutes	Stretch: 2 minutes		

Remember, walking on Tuesdays and over weekends is optional to start with, as you get used to your new walking program.

WEEK FOUR

Week four of the beginner program sees a five-minute increase of your daily walking time and Tuesdays are no longer optional. Try for a walking pace of 3 to 3.5 miles per hour. Try to start including one day over the weekend.

Monday	Tuesday	Wednesday	Thursday	Friday	Weekends
Warm up: 1 minute	Warm up: 1 minute	Warm up: 1 minute	Warm up: 1 minute	Rest	Warm up: 1 minute
Stretch: 2 minutes	Stretch: 2 minutes	Stretch: 2 minutes	Stretch: 2 minutes		Stretch: 2 minutes
Easy walk: 10 minutes	Easy walk: 10 - 15 minutes	Easy walk: 10 minutes	Easy walk 10 - 15 minutes		Easy walk: 10 - 15 minutes
Brisk walk: 5 minutes	Stretch: 2 minutes	Brisk walk: 5 minutes	Stretch: 2 minutes		Stretch: 2 minutes
Stretch: 2 minutes		Stretch: 2 minutes			

WEEK FIVE

Another 5-minute increase of your daily walking time is in store for you in week five. Try for a walking pace of 3 to 3.5 miles per hour. Try to start including one day over the weekend.

Monday	Tuesday	Wednesday	Thursday	Friday	Weekends
Warm up: 1 minute	Warm up: 1 minute	Warm up: 1 minute	Warm up: 1 minute	Rest	Warm up: 1 minute
Stretch: 2 minutes	Stretch: 2 minutes	Stretch: 2 minutes	Stretch: 2 minutes		Stretch: 2 minutes
Easy walk: 10 - 15 minutes	Easy walk: 15 - 20 minutes	Easy walk: 10 - 15 minutes	Easy walk: 15 - 20 minutes		Easy walk: 15 - 20 minutes
Brisk walk: 5 - 10 minutes	Stretch: 2 minutes	Brisk walk: 5 - 10 minutes	Stretch: 2 minutes		Stretch: 2 minutes
Stretch: 2 minutes		Stretch: 2 minutes			

WEEK SIX

You guessed it, increase your walking time by another 5 minutes. Try for a walking pace of 3 to 3.5 miles per hour. Include one day over the weekend.

Monday	Tuesday	Wednesday	Thursday	Friday	Weekends
Warm up: 1 minute	Warm up: 1 minute	Warm up: 1 minute	Warm up: 1 minute	Rest	Warm up: 1 minute
Stretch: 2 minutes	Stretch: 2 minutes	Stretch: 2 minutes	Stretch: 2 minutes		Stretch: 2 minutes
Brisk walk: 25 minutes	Easy walk or an alternative activity of your choice: 20 - 25 minutes	Brisk walk: 25 minutes	Brisk walk: 25 minutes		Brisk walk: 25 minutes
Stretch: 2 minutes	Stretch: 2 minutes	Stretch: 2 minutes	Stretch: 2 minutes		Stretch: 2 minutes

WEEK SEVEN

Tack on that last 5 minutes in week seven to reach a total walking time of 30 minutes. Try for a walking pace of 3 to 3.5 miles per hour (or faster if you can manage). Include one day over the weekend.

Monday	Tuesday	Wednesday	Thursday	Friday	Weekends
Warm up: 1 minute	Warm up: 1 minute	Warm up: 1 minute	Warm up: 1 minute	Rest	Warm up: 1 minute
Stretch: 2 minutes	Stretch: 2 minutes	Stretch: 2 minutes	Stretch: 2 minutes		Stretch: 2 minutes
Brisk walk: 30 minutes	Easy walk or an alternative activity of your choice: 20 - 30 minutes	Brisk walk: 30 minutes	Brisk walk: 30 minutes		Brisk walk: 30 minutes
Stretch: 2 minutes	Stretch: 2 minutes	Stretch: 2 minutes	Stretch: 2 minutes		Stretch: 2 minutes

TAKING YOUR WALKING PROGRAM FURTHER

After week seven, you can work your way up to an intermediate level of walking. You can do this by following the intermediate guidelines above. Additional tips include:

- Continue to increase your walking time by 5 - 10 minutes per week.
- If you cannot extend your walking time, increase your pace.

- If you increase your walking time, but can't sustain an increased pace for the whole walk, walk in intervals of slower and faster pace until you can walk at a faster pace for the whole walk.
- If you can increase your pace for the whole walk, but can't sustain the increased pace for every walk of the week, try alternating between an increased pace for one walk and a slower pace for the next, etc.

Once you are ready to move on to a more advanced walking level, try following the advanced guidelines in chapter 2. You can also:

- Continue to gradually increase your pace to a power-walking pace. If you are already at a power-walking pace and feel up to increasing the pace further, try alternating between power walking and a slow jog in intervals. (Consult your doctor before including a slow jog pace, especially if you have past injuries or joint trouble.)
- Take short breaks from walking to alternate between walking and doing bodyweight exercises such as lunges, squats, press-ups, etc.

WALKING OUTDOORS

One of the best ways to naturally challenge yourself and increase the efficacy of your walking for weight loss fitness program is to take your walking outdoors. Yes, a treadmill is a great thing and it has a time and a place. However, there is much more you can enjoy and take advantage of when you walk outdoors. In the next chapter, we're going to tell you why you should walk outdoors and the different ways you can walk outside.

4

THE ULTIMATE GUIDE TO OUTDOOR WALKING

Walking outdoors is immensely rewarding and offers a variety of benefits over just stepping onto a treadmill. It's not just weight loss that will be a benefit received from walking outdoors. It will create a happier, healthier you through improving your holistic health, including mental and emotional well-being. Let's take a look at the various benefits and types of outdoor walking you can take advantage of.

BENEFITS OF WALKING OUTDOORS

Walking outdoors has the same benefits as walking indoors or anywhere else as far as your physical health is concerned but it has a few aces up its sleeve as an added bonus. Walking outdoors offers walkers these added benefits.

Get Some Fresh Air

There is a common saying in stressful situations; people often say they are going to 'get some fresh air'. This phrase was coined for a reason. Getting outside, out of the stuffiness of indoors, makes you feel better but why?

Oxygen; the simple answer is oxygen. It helps your brain function better, heal from damage such as free radicals, and even grow. Brain function is influenced by oxygen levels and we all know those aren't always stellar indoors. Getting outside for a walk gives you a chance to breathe in more oxygen for happier, healthier 'mental muscle'.

Reduce Your Stress

It's suggested that spending a lot of time indoors can contribute to your stress levels while getting enough outdoor time among green scenery can help alleviate stress. When you take a walk outside to 'get some fresh air' part of that feel-good effect is that your brain produces the mood-regulating neurotransmitters, endorphins. They are essentially your good-mood chemicals in your brain. Essentially, walking outdoors is like a dose of natural therapy that can reduce your stress, thereby reducing your negative thoughts, and create a happier, healthier emotional and mental state.

More Vitamin D

Your body can only make vitamin D when your skin is exposed to sunlight. Vitamin D is an essential nutrient your brain needs to function. It has been suggested that this vitamin reduces inflammation in the brain, offers neuron protection, and even helps your brain make neurotransmitters and aids in nerve growth. A sedentary lifestyle is typically lived indoors, away from sunlight, so getting outdoors for your walk provides you with a healthy dose of sunshine.

TYPES OF OUTDOOR WALKING

Some types of outdoor walking are better suited for more rugged, natural terrain while others require a more structured natural approach like city parks and urban green spaces. When you think about walking outdoors, you probably conjure up a mental image of hiking in majestic mountainous areas, but that's not where the possibilities end. Walking outdoors simply means getting out of the house or office. The more natural the setting you are walking in, the better. However, you can easily take your walking to a nearby urban park or green area for a variety of different types and styles of walking to switch up your routine and bust boredom.

Hiking

If you are not used to hiking, even if you aren't a complete novice walker, it can seem like a daunting task. Long, hard trails up steep mountainsides may come to mind. While that is a *cookie cutter* idea of hiking, it's not necessarily the case. Hiking comes in all shapes and sizes, from short, gentle trails for beginners to long, challenging trails for the more experienced. You can find a trail to suit your needs and experience level, so don't worry about that.

The beauty of hiking is, well, the beauty. It gets you out there, into the great outdoors. From easy forest trails to breathtaking mountain ranges, there is something stunning and natural to be found on every trail. The fresh air, combined with beautiful natural scenery, has a feel-good effect that can make hiking seem more like a day out in nature than a walking workout. Despite the challenge of different terrains, you will probably enjoy your time hiking much more than pounding the pavements or paved walkways in parks.

Speaking of terrain, hiking naturally mixes things up by offering a wide variety of terrains in a single walk. There will be level sections, inclines, slopes, solid ground, mud after rain, and even soft, sandy patches. Why is this a bonus for your walk? Each different terrain presents its own unique challenges to your body, working with different muscles. If you've ever walked on a soft, sandy beach, you know just how much more of a sweat you can work up and the different muscles used versus walking on level concrete.

Beginner Hiking Tips

If you aren't a seasoned hiker, you shouldn't just head out to hit the trails without some planning and preparation. Here are some tips for getting started if you're a newcomer to the wondrous world of hiking.

Make the Right Trail Choice

Choosing the right trail for your skill level and the right distance for your fitness level is incredibly important to prevent injury and discouragement.

- Research different trails, their lengths, and rated difficulty levels.
- Choose a trail shorter than the distance you can walk on paved or level ground.
- Estimate an average hiking pace of two miles per hour, even if you can walk faster on a paved or level surface.
- Tack on an hour extra to your overall estimated time for every 1,000 feet of elevation gain.

Get Familiar

- After choosing your trail, do your research.
- Consult maps of the area and online resources.
- Determine if the trail is a thoroughfare from one road to another, a loop, or if it dead ends and you'll have to double back.
- Make notes of where trails intersect to avoid making a wrong turn.
- Determine good rest spots.

Tell Someone

To avoid panicking friends and family and to make search and rescue quicker and easier if required, tell someone where you will be. Include the following in your information:

- The area you are going to.
- The trail you have chosen.
- When you will start.
- What your general itinerary is.

Be sure to leave enough time for wiggle room before they should start worrying, in case of delays such as hiking slower than anticipated or stopping to take in the view.

Tip: A portable emergency tracking device can be used to call for help if you get into trouble while hiking. Don't rely solely on a tracking device though. Always tell someone where you are going.

What's the Weather?

- Check the weather a few days before and again a few hours before your hike.
- Decide what to pack and how to dress, based on the forecast.
- Don't hit the trail if the weather is forecasted to turn foul mid-hike.

Clothing Choice

Aside from picking out the right footwear, your clothing choice will affect your comfort and enjoyment.

- Steer clear of cotton, as it absorbs moisture and can cause chafing.
- Opt for synthetic materials.
- Wear a moisture-wicking base layer to keep sweat away from your body.
- Wear light layers that can be added or stripped off, according to temperature changes.
- Take one more warm layer, which blocks wind, than you think you need.

Footwear

- Use the shoe-buying tips previously provided to find the best hiking boot fit.
- Choose shoes that are water- and mud-resistant. Wet shoes, socks, and feet aren't fun.
- Choose synthetic or wool socks, no cotton.

Tip: Throw blister dressings into your backpack, just in case.

Ten Must-Have Essentials

Expect the best, but prepare for the worst. Being prepared can be a life-saver and make you feel more confident.

1. Emergency shelter (an emergency tent of some sort; even a garbage bag can do the trick).
2. Extra water.
3. Fire (waterproof matches/lighter).
4. First-aid kit.
5. Light (flashlight/headlamp).
6. Extra clothing (not the additional, wind-resistant, layer mentioned above).
7. Navigation (map and compass).
8. Extra food.
9. Compact repair kit and tools.
10. Sun protection (sunscreen and eye protection).

Light Load

Choose the lightest-weight option for each of the 10 essentials. For example, pack a compact first aid kit and travel-sized sunscreen.

Pace Perfect

Pace yourself so that you don't empty the tank before you reach the end of your hike. Feeling strong and energetic at the start can fool you into tackling the trail full steam ahead; resist the temptation.

No Trace Left Behind

There is a quote that perfectly sums up the attitude you should cultivate to preserve the world's natural spaces.

> "Take only memories. Leave only footprints."
>
> — CHIEF SEATTLE

OTHER TYPES OF OUTDOOR WALKING

As we've said, hiking isn't the only type of walking you can enjoy outdoors. Here's a rundown of other types and styles of walking you can try outdoors to make your walking routine more interesting and up your calorie burn.

Brisk Walking

Different people walk briskly at different speeds depending on their fitness level. A rule of thumb is around 100 steps per minute or 3.5 miles per hour. Benefits include a higher heart rate than regular walking and an increased calorie burn.

Stroller Walking

Got young kids? There's no excuse for you to stay cooped up indoors. New moms and dads can get outdoors, take the kids with them, and enjoy working out as a family. Many strollers will do the job, but there are some specialized strollers available.

Power Walking

The pace of power walking is higher than brisk walking, but just less than a jog. Swing your arms vigorously while power walking for a full-body workout. Aim for 4 to 5.5 miles per hour. Nailing that heel-to-toe technique mentioned earlier and a 90-degree arm swing is the key to success.

Tip: To make power walking more effective, add ankle and wrist weights once you get the hang of it.

Nordic Walking (Pole Walking)

Nordic walking increases the pace and helps with inclines, uneven surfaces, and balance. It offers the walker a full-body workout by using poles to engage the upper body and propel them forward. The pace to walk at is brisk to power walking.

Race Walking

A competitive sport, even an Olympic event, race walking takes walking speed to the extreme. Race walking offers a high-intensity workout and ramps up the calorie burn. It is characterized by:

- One foot always being in contact with the ground.
- Shorter strides.
- Straight-legged walking style with a pronounced side-to-side hip rotation.

Marathon Walking

You've heard about marathon running. Now, we're going to tell you about marathon walking. Distance average 26.2 miles or 42.195 kilometers with a general time limit of six hours. The focus of marathon walkers is maintaining a steady speed to increase endurance. Training usually starts nine months prior to a race and consists of a single long walk per week that gradually increases to cover the full distance as well as the walker's regular walking workout schedule.

Chi Walking

Chi walking concentrates on walking form to improve posture, relax muscles, increase core strength, and improve cardio fitness. Employing mindfulness helps walkers focus on proper alignment of the body by using Thai Chi principles to not only work the body, but also involve the mind and spirit.

WALKING STYLES EXPLAINED

Some of the walking styles mentioned above need some further explanation to understand and make proper use of.

Stroller Walking

Stroller walking is a great way to combine family time and get your walking workout in at the same time. The added bonus is encouraging little ones to enjoy the outdoors and planting the seed about the importance of a healthy, active lifestyle. This is especially important in our age of modern technology which is causing children to spend less time outdoors and more time being sedentary indoors while glued to their tech toys.

Your Stroller Matters

Many regular strollers might do the trick for a casual stroll. A specialized exercise stroller will make a difference to a dedicated walking parent who wants to make the most of their walk. Advantages include better wheels for improved baby comfort and more handle height adjustments to accommodate handle height for a better stride.

What should you look for in an exercise stroller?

- Easy locking brakes for additional activities such as lunging.
- Quality covers with vents for breathability and protecting your child from sun exposure.
- Various reclining positions to accommodate your little one's desire to be more active or lie down for a nap.
- Easy manoeuvrability for paths that are not straight.

Posture

An extendable handle will help you to maintain better posture. Stroller walking can lead to poor posture, so you need to mind your posture while doing so.

- Engage your core (abdominal muscles).
- Maintain a neutral wrist position.
- Keep your head up and your shoulders back and down.
- Keep your hips and the stroller close together.
- Try using the stroller in a one-handed grip and alternating your arm swinging to get your upper body moving and ward off stiffness.

Routes

- Hot days require a more shaded path.
- Smooth surfaces are optimal. Hiking trails aren't a good choice.
- Paths and parks meant for use by multiple users are better than single tracks.
- Safety.
- Always engage the breaks when you take both hands off the handle.
- Take walks in neighborhoods you're familiar with.
- Avoid busy streets.
- Let someone know where you're going to be walking and keep your phone handy in case of an emergency.

Additional Stroller Walking Workout

Warm-Up: Walk for five minutes at an easy pace to warm your muscles. Roll your shoulders and perform ankle rotations as detailed previously.

Intervals: Alternate walking as quickly as possible with 30 seconds of slower-paced walking to recover and catch your breath. Repeat five times. You should feel the muscle effort and be breathing hard from the exertion.

Chest Press Single-Arm: Use an incline and your stroller in front of you. Hold onto the handle with one hand, arm bent at the elbow. Push the stroller away from you and pull it back toward you. Perform 12 reps with each arm.

Walking Lunge: Work your glutes, hamstrings, and quads all at once. Take a big step forward with one foot, planting your forward foot firmly on the ground. Bend both knees. Your back knee will move toward the ground. Make sure your forward knee doesn't move forward past your toes as it bends. Your front knee should bend to approximately 90 degrees or until your thigh is parallel to the ground. Press down through your feet to come fully upright before taking another walking lunge with the other foot. Chest out and back straight through the movement. Perform walking lunges for three minutes.

Power Walk: For five minutes, use full strides to slowly increase intensity. Increase the intensity each minute to reach a challenging pace by the end.

Cool Down: Walk slowly for five minutes to recover, bringing your breathing and heart rate back down.

Reverse Curl: Park your stroller on a soft surface, brakes engaged. Lie on your back in front of the stroller, with your head positioned at the front wheels. Bring your hands over your head, taking hold of the footrest or one wheel. Bend your knees until your legs create a 90-degree angle. Squeeze and contract your core abdominal muscles, tilting your pelvis to bring your legs slightly toward you. Perform three sets of 15 repetitions each.

Crunches: Using the same soft surface, turn around and lie on your back with your feet at the base of the stroller or the footrest. Bend your knees to a 45-degree angle and clasp your hands behind your head. Don't pull your head forward as you perform a traditional crunch so you come off the ground only up to your shoulders. Perform three sets of 15 repetitions each.

Stretching: You should perform these stretches after your warmup and cool down.

Hamstring Stretch: Place your right foot on the wheel, holding onto the handle with your left hand, brakes engaged. Place your right hand on your right thigh and sit back into the stretch by leaning your upper body forward and pushing your hips back. You should feel the stretch in the back of your left thigh. Repeat with both legs.

Hip Stretch: Perform the hip stretch detailed previously while holding onto the handle with both hands, brakes engaged. Repeat with both legs.

Calf Stretch: Place your hand on the handle, brakes engaged. Put your right toe against the right wheel, leaning your body forward and keeping your heel on the ground. Lean forward and feel the stretch in your calf muscle. Repeat with both legs.

NORDIC WALKING

Nordic walking is easily accessible to walkers and doesn't require a specific type of terrain and very little equipment not already needed for general walking. It enhances your walking by giving you an increased pace and uses your upper body for a total body workout.

The Gear

- Nordic walking poles are the only additional equipment you need to get started.
- Be sure to purchase the specialized Nordic walking poles, which have necessary accessories such as interchangeable attachments for different terrains and correct hand straps.
- Regular ski poles are not suitable.
- Purchase poles suitable for your walking stride and height. Adjustable and fixed poles are available.

- Pole height should only be long enough to be held vertically while your elbows are bent at a 90-degree angle.
- If purchasing adjustable poles, have them correctly fitted before exiting the store.
- Wrist straps are recommended, but not strictly necessary.
- Wrist straps look like the bottom cuffs of gloves and fit around the thumbs.
- Choose comfortable straps which allow release on the backstroke and return to the right position on the forward stroke.
- Attachable rubber pads for pavement walking should come as part of the purchase, but always make sure to get them.
- Walking on dirt utilizes the metal spike.
- Regular walking shoes are suitable for pavement walking.
- Hiking shoes are used for *off road* terrain.
- Refer to the walking shoe purchasing guide in the first chapter to purchase shoes.

Nordic Walking Techniques

- Properly strap the poles to your wrists via the straps.
- Begin by walking normally.
- Don't use the poles, but hold them lightly.

- Natural gait is used for Nordic walking. It's important to maintain your natural gait and arm swing.
- As you advance, walking faster will naturally lengthen your stride.
- Using a heel-to-toe stepping motion, you will plant the pole opposite to your forward foot onto the ground and propel your body forward with a push. If you step forward with your right foot, plant the pole with your left hand.
- Allow the poles to be pulled along behind you, angled at 45 degrees.
- When the angle is correct, plant the poles into the ground at that angle. You will maintain a 45-degree angle while walking.
- Keep your elbows tucked close to your body, arms relaxed and straight.
- Start applying more pressure with each push to achieve a fuller arm swing as you get comfortable.
- Keep the poles planted and pushing as you take a step with your other foot, keeping your arms in motion.
- Maintain straight hips and head, ensuring that your torso rotates slightly with each step, as it would when walking normally. Your torso should rotate slightly to the left when you step forward with your right foot and vice versa when stepping with the left foot.

- Begin walking short distances, for about 30 minutes, to avoid excessive muscle soreness.
- Extend walking time and distance as your body adjusts.
- Nordic walking uses more muscles than regular walking, increasing calorie burn by up to 46 percent.

Workout Advancement

When you are ready to advance your Nordic walking workout, here's how to do it:

- Walk at a normal pace during your first walk. Don't try to speed off into the distance just yet.
- Focus on technique and form to get it right.
- On the second day, extend your walk to 50 minutes, alternating between longer and normal strides every 15 minutes which mimics HIIT.
- Stop if it doesn't feel comfortable. Decrease intensity if necessary.
- Walk normally for 30 minutes on the third day. Walking without poles now and then helps maintain your natural walking style. It also allows your body some rest from Nordic walking.
- On the fourth day, progress to rolling terrain and extend the walk to 60 minutes. Practice both uphill and downhill walking. Pace yourself.
- Take a 40-minute walk on the fifth day, paying attention to posture.

- Do not walk at all on the sixth day, allowing your body to rest and recover.
- On the seventh day of the week, aim for a 75-minute walk. Make use of trails as much as possible.
- When 75-minute walks are comfortable, you can increase your walk time by 15 minutes per week.

RACE WALKING

Race walking is a very specific, learned technique that is not a natural body movement for walking.

Getting Ready

Always warm up by walking easily and stretching for 5 to 10 minutes.

Race Walking Technique

Correct form is the key to successful race walking and preventing injury. Here's how to do race walking correctly:

Head Position

- Maintain a relaxed jaw and neck.
- Maintain a level head, with eyes focused about 20 yards ahead.

Arms

- Always maintain a bend at the elbows of 85 to 90 degrees.
- Swing your arms vigorously from the shoulders. Keep your arms loose.
- Hands are held close to the body, brushing hip bones with the heels of your hands.
- Your hands should not come up higher horizontally than the middle of your torso or come across further vertically than the middle.
- At the end of swinging your arm upward, your upper arm should be vertically in line with your torso so that you don't bring your hands upward.
- When swinging your arms backward, imagine that you are reaching for your hip pockets.
- Do not swing past your range of motion which could result in restriction of breathing and a forward, bent-over posture.
- Clench your fist loosely, thumb on top, but always maintain relaxed hands.

Torso

- Walk up straight and keep your body relaxed.
- Don't lean forward or push your tush out backward.
- Engage your core muscles, keeping the curvature of your lower back neutral.

- A completely relaxed core could cause what is called *sway back*.
- Prevent tensing your neck and shoulders by keeping your shoulders relaxed.

Hips

- Rotate the pelvis horizontally back and forth like you would if you were dancing the 60's Twist.
- You will be twisting using the side abdominal muscles.
- To prevent injury to the muscles on the sides of your hips and glutes, avoid moving your hips overly from side to side.
- To help maintain a proper hip twist, drive the knees forward toward the center of your body.

Legs and Stride

- Keep the knee of the leg moving forward straight, but not locked, as it hits the ground.
- Bend the knee as little as possible when swinging your leg forward.
- Begin by walking slowly. Increase the pace as you go along.
- Maintain your body's natural stride length as you increase the pace to avoid overstriding. Aim for around 160 steps per minute. You may even progress

to between 180 and 200 steps with practice and experience.
- Stride length may initially become shorter as you increase the pace.

Feet

- One foot must always be in contact with the ground. The front foot must touch the ground before lifting the back foot.
- The key to race walking is a short stride. Putting your forward foot down too far ahead of your upper body lengthens the stride, slows your pace, and could result in groin injury and what is known as *soft knee*. Overstriding can also injure the glutes and hamstrings on inclines.
- Use a heel-to-toe stepping motion, flexing the ankle as your foot strikes the ground and straightening it before lifting it off the ground. Lifting a flexed ankle could cause tendon injury.
- Keep the ankle relaxed as you bring your leg forward to take a step, pointing your toes at the ground until your foot has passed the leg you are standing on. Begin flexing the ankle once past the supporting leg.
- Ease into race walking until the muscles get used to this to prevent tightness, soreness, and burning.

Race Walking Rules and Mistakes

- You will be disqualified if the knee of the leg moving forward is not straight from the moment it touches the ground, through the lift, until it passes the supporting leg.
- Avoid leaning either forward or backward. Maintain a straight body as much as possible. Leaning backward slows you down and makes maintaining a straight leg difficult.
- You will receive a lift violation or might be disqualified if one foot is not in contact with the ground at all times.
- Avoid overstriding, a common mistake in both regular and race walking. Focus on keeping the forward motion of your leading leg shorter, but the backward motion of the leg pushing you forward slightly longer for a powerful push.
- Use powerful arm motions to counteract the leg and hip twist, but don't cross the midlines of your torso, either horizontally or vertically.
- Elbows should not rock side-to-side, but rather move in a more back-and-forth motion.

Important note: As well as reading these instructions, watch videos, attend a race walking clinic, or get professional coaching. Poor techniques could result in a loss of speed and efficiency as well as injury.

CHI WALKING

Chi walking is a gentle yet effective style of walking that will not only help you melt away the pounds, but also improve posture, muscle strength, and flexibility. Chi walking is a mindful connection between the mind and body while providing you with a good daily dose of walking exercise. Here's how to get started with chi walking:

Alignment

- Align yourself physically and mentally by using mindfulness to ground yourself and bring you into the present.
- Feel your body, noticing your posture.
- Feel the ground under your feet, how your muscles feel, and how the breeze or sunshine feels on your skin. Be fully present in your body and feel every sensation there is to feel.
- Pay attention to your posture, and stand up straight and tall with your feet shoulder-width apart.
- Imagine dots on your ankles, hips, and shoulders, with a straight invisible line running upwards, connecting them together.
- Aligning your body will take the stress off your muscles and allow your bones to support you.
- Imagine drawing your energy to the vertical centerline up your spine while relaxing your arms

and legs. All of your movement will come from this strong centerline.

Engage Your Core

- Allow your feet and knees to relax. Feel your knee go soft, but not wobbly.
- Elongate your spine as if you are a puppet with a string attached to the top of your head. Feel that string being pulled gently upward and your spine lengthening.
- Level your pelvis by making sure your weight is evenly distributed between both legs.
- Put one hand on your abdomen, placing your fingers just above your pelvic bone and your thumb at your belly button.
- Engage your pelvic muscles and feel them under your fingers. Feel how activating those muscles pulls your pelvis gently upward, but not too far.
- Imagine a bowl of water inside your pelvis. Level it out so that water doesn't spill over the front or back.

Create Balance

- Create balance by making sure that you maintain your body weight over your leading foot. Remember that all movement comes from that strong center line.

- Your core muscles should be doing the majority of the work when you move; not your legs and feet pulling you along with them.
- Physical balance helps prevent falls by keeping you centered.
- Make the choice to move forward differently from the way you have always done.
- You are going to lead with your upper body instead of your feet.
- Choose the direction you will move in before you start moving to bring all parts of your body into unison to move together as one.

Move Forward

- Moving forward means more than just taking a step forward. It can be extended to your whole life.
- Moving forward in chi walking means making a deliberate and conscious decision to take a step and to commit to today's walk as well as your walking plan for the week. You are not just moving, you are moving toward weight loss, health, and happiness.
- Maintain mindfulness of your posture, engaged core, and balance while moving forward.
- Keep your goal in mind.
- Take four steps forward and ensure that your movement is balanced and has both direction and purpose before continuing.

Chi walking is about more than just walking. It is about synchronizing your body and mind. It is about intention and direction, not only on the walking path, but also in life. Remain aware of what is going on around you while you walk, but also maintain mindfulness of your body and mind.

Important note: Chi walking is a great form of moving meditation that requires practice to get your body and mind in the same space. If you are interested in taking up Chi walking, look up some how-to videos for more information and *hands-on* step-by-step instructions.

MAKE WALKING FUN

Walking is a great way to explore the world and see things you have always overlooked from behind the wheel or in the passenger seat of a car. You also get to experience more of your surroundings more deeply; breathing in the fresh air, feeling the breeze, and hearing the sounds. If that isn't enough to keep you entertained, try making your walks even more fun or meaningful with a few simple activities.

Photography

Everybody has a smartphone these days and the camera technology you hold in the palm of your hand is perfect for becoming a walking shutterbug. Don't just plug your earphones in and switch on your tunes; use your phone to maximize your walking experience and make memories.

Street and landscape photography is a great way to really see what is going on around you. It will also allow your creativity to go wild. The best part is, you will probably be so busy looking for photo opportunities that you won't even be aware of just how far you're actually walking.

Moving Meditation

Meditation is often seen as a stationary or sedentary practice. You sit, you close your eyes, and you meditate. However, you don't have to confine yourself to seated meditation. Get your body moving and bring stillness to your mind at the same time with walking meditation.

As you walk, direct your focus and attention to your feet. Feel how every part of your foot feels throughout the process of taking each step. Focus on every aspect of the sensations you feel from how your foot feels in your shoe to how it feels as it flexes and moves.

You will probably need to walk a bit slower than usual when you first start. Really get the feel of your feet, as you can speed up later or use moving meditation for a few minutes during or after your walk to help manage stress.

It may feel awkward in the beginning. Our minds aren't used to being quiet and focused on one thing. We are so used to having dozens of thoughts flit through our heads and loads of distractions intrude that creating a sense of stillness can seem difficult. The key to success is understanding that it's not about completely clearing your head of all thoughts. What you are doing is teaching yourself that you don't have to pay attention to every thought that pops into your head. Your mind will stray off to what you're having for dinner or whether you sent that important email. What you need to do is retrieve your attention and refocus it back onto your feet, calming your mind again. Over time, this will become easier and easier until you reach a meditative state during your walking meditation sessions.

Geocaching

Have you heard about geocaching? If not, get ready to have some fun on your walks. Geocaching has taken the world by storm with millions of geocaches hidden all over the globe. You never know; there might even be some near you right now.

Geocaching is kind of like a high-tech game of treasure hunting. Caches are containers that are hidden in various locations. Using a geocaching app on your mobile phone, you can use the GPS coordinates of these hidden caches to find them. Within each container is usually a logbook or log sheet you can sign or some other way of registering that you found the cache. Can you think of a better way to get your daily steps in than playing a giant hidden treasure game?

WALKING INDOORS

There is nothing like walking outdoors. It is one of the best spaces to walk in. However, there are a variety of reasons why you may not be able to get outside to meet your walking fitness program needs. In the next chapter, we'll cover the different ways you can fit walking into your time spent indoors and how to make a workout of it when you don't have a treadmill.

5

INDOOR WALKING: DON'T LET THE WEATHER PUT YOU OFF

Spending time in the great outdoors on your walking for weight loss journey is incredibly beneficial to your overall health and well-being. However, there are times when the weather doesn't want to play ball, making it difficult for you to get outdoors for your walks. There are also times you are inevitably stuck indoors for extended periods of time, such as while working from home, etc. This may seem like a deterrent to sticking with your regime, but it's not. Walking outdoors is awesome, but including indoor spaces broadens your scope of walking possibilities so that you get the most out of your walking program.

INDOOR WALKING BENEFITS

Walking indoors offers most of the same benefits as taking walks outdoors. Aside from the advantages of fresh air, vitamin D, and the inherent relaxation that comes from walking outdoors, walking indoors will offer you all the same health and weight loss benefits. However, keeping it indoors does have a few advantages of its own.

Weather is not a factor when you are walking indoors. If it's hot outside and you have the option of walking indoors, you won't feel like you're melting as you pound the pavement. If your area is experiencing inclement weather, you can stay warm and toasty while walking indoors, instead of feeling like a walking human popsicle.

Wear what you want without any considerations. When you take your walks outdoors, you have to give several considerations to your outfit choice.

- Will you need layers for changes in temperature?
- Will the color of your walking clothes absorb more heat in cold weather or reflect heat in hot weather?
- If it's warmer, will you have to slather on sunscreen to protect your skin from sun exposure?

When walking indoors, you don't have to worry about any of these things. You can wear whatever you want to wear that makes you feel good while you're walking.

Walking indoors typically throws fewer challenges your way. Walking outdoors presents you with variables such as insects, exposure to the weather, avoiding both vehicular and pedestrian traffic which could slow or interfere with your walking efforts, and coming across animals. Staying indoors from time to time minimizes those challenges and lets you get on with what's important; putting all your effort and focus into your exertion, time, and distance.

Walking indoors keeps things consistent. When you walk outdoors, there are many things that could change from day to day, including traffic, weather, and even the route you take. Switching things up is a great way to stave off boredom, but it can make achieving consistent results more difficult.

CONSIDERATIONS FOR WALKING INDOORS

Walking indoors can make achieving your walking for weight loss goals more convenient at times, especially when it comes to bad weather days. However, before you embark on indoor walking sessions, there are a few things to consider.

Safety

Yes, walking indoors can be a safer option than taking a walk outside, but that doesn't mean it's an inherently safe practice. There are a few safety precautions to bear in mind when walking indoors:

- Ensure that you know how to properly and safely operate any walking-related fitness equipment you will be using. This includes treadmills, steppers, etc., and how to work their emergency shutdown buttons if needed.
- Ensure that all staircases you plan to use have properly secured hand railings in case you suddenly need the support.

Equipment

Walking indoors technically doesn't require any equipment at all. That being said, if you do have equipment available to you, you can use as much or as little of it as you want to. If you are thinking of investing in indoor walking equipment, take your available space and budget into account when making a decision.

Tip: Invest in a basic, but high-quality pedometer to help you track your steps indoors if you can't easily measure the distance. Walking pace can vary, even if you think you are putting the same amount of effort into maintaining speed. So, measuring your walking workout on time alone can be a bit misleading and a pedometer will help take some of that uncertainty out of it.

Accessibility

How accessible is your preferred indoor walking space? You may need to find several indoor walking spaces to accommodate changes in routine and whether that space has opening hours or not. Walking inside your own home offers you 24-hour access, but a shopping mall has set opening hours and your work office building is only available on the days you work. Think about a variety of different options to offer you walking access as often as possible when you need to walk indoors.

OPTIONS FOR WALKING INDOORS

The first thing that comes to mind when thinking of ways to walk indoors is a treadmill. While this is a convenient option, it's not your only option. You have a variety of indoor walking methods to take advantage of, depending on accessibility.

Treadmill

The most obvious option, a treadmill, is easy to use and offers adjustments such as increasing pace and adding inclines. You can even program it to alternate between different inclines and flats to simulate an outdoor workout with varying terrain. Additional benefits of using a treadmill include safety from traffic, other people, and animals, a lack of obstacles, and you certainly won't get lost. When you can focus purely on your walking, you can concentrate on developing good walking posture.

The drawback of walking on a treadmill is that you may become bored. There is no change of scenery and it's generally something you'll do alone. When it comes to walking on a treadmill, technology is your best friend. You can listen to music, podcasts, audiobooks, follow a live-streamed treadmill workout, or even watch your favorite TV shows.

Buying a treadmill requires certain considerations:

- Quality.
- Available space. If you lack the space for a standard treadmill, a folding treadmill may be an option.
- Adjustments and features to enhance your walking workout.
- Stability.
- The power of the motor.

Walking In a Mall

Yes, mall walking is a thing. It's a great balance between exercise and being social, plus you get to window shop at the same time. Malls are also a safe space to walk and offer conveniences such as restrooms and access to food and beverages if you need them.

Malls are a good option for slower walks and while you can walk with friends or other mall walkers, obstacles are aplenty. You'll have to navigate between shoppers, store aisles and displays, benches, etc.

Important note: Malls have hard concrete floors, so opt for a walking shoe with more cushioning to absorb the impact.

Walking in an Airport

Travelling can see you sitting for long hours at a time, especially on long-distance flights. A new development in some airports is the introduction of designated walking paths within the terminal. You can stretch your legs, get your body moving, and get those steps in toward your 10,000-step goal instead of sitting around waiting for your flight.

In the U.S., walker-friendly airports include:

- Cleveland Hopkins International Airport (CLE).
- Dallas-Fort Worth International Airport (DFW).
- Minneapolis-St. Paul International Airport (MSP).
- Phoenix Sky Harbor International Airport (PHX).
- Thurgood Marshall Airport (BWI).

Create an Indoor Walking Circuit

You can get creative at school or at work by creating your own walking circuit. Large buildings offer a variety of hallways and even stairs to help you get your steps in and vary the intensity. If you want some company while walking, start a walking group for other walkers to join in. Not only will you be getting your steps in, but you can make new friends and catch up on what's going on around the school or workplace.

Tip: Whenever possible, take the stairs instead of the elevator at work or school to maximize your daily walking.

Guided Video Walking Workouts

Guided walking workouts are available online and on DVD. You can utilize these workouts without a treadmill and with limited indoor space. These walking workout videos help you tone muscles and burn calories while making use of exercises such as marching in place, knee lifts, kicks, and side steps.

Video walking workouts are freely available online through video websites such as YouTube. When it comes to picking a great workout, two names to look out for are Jessica Smith and Leslie Sansone. These women present workouts that will get you moving and improve balance, strength, flexibility, and coordination all in one workout.

Important note: Video walking workouts are not a substitute for outdoor walking training when preparing for a long walk such as a walking marathon event.

Indoor Walking Tracks

Indoor running and walking tracks are available at some health facilities and gyms. These are safe, indoor spaces dedicated to offering walkers the opportunity to get their steps in away from distractions, obstacles, and inclement weather. These tracks often have lanes set up, so it's important that you don't block other walkers or runners and follow the direction and lane rules of the track. The bonus is that you can time yourself effectively, walk in alternating intervals, and increase your pace by trying to catch up to other walkers. However, due to the rules, indoor walking tracks aren't a good place for walking with a group of friends.

WALKING AT HOME

You don't have to live in a mansion to add steps to your day. You can make up a big chunk of your daily steps in any size home by switching things up in a few simple ways. This is especially useful if you work from home.

Get a Smartwatch

Even more useful than a pedometer, a smartwatch has more features such as reminders to move when it detects that you've been inactive for a set period of time. You don't have to fork out for the latest and greatest smartwatch. Do some online research and comparisons to find a watch that has the features you need and will make use of.

Reminders are a great way to prompt you to get up and walk, especially if you work from home and get lost in what you are doing. You can also earn digital rewards, which may sound silly at first, but can be useful as motivation to pay attention to your watch when it tells you to get moving.

Note: Read more about smartwatches and activity tracking in Chapter 7.

Cook on the Move

Making your daily step goal doesn't restrict you to only walking. Have some fun in the kitchen and multitask. If marching in place isn't your thing, make it more fun by dancing around the kitchen. Every step you take is a step, irrespective of how you take that step. Even if you're not cooking up a storm, dance, march in place, or pace up and down while you wait for the kettle to boil, food to reheat in the microwave, or the toaster to pop up. Pretty much anything that leaves you waiting around in the kitchen presents an opportunity for movement. Every step counts, even if you're only moving for a minute or two at a time.

Phone Walking

Working from home has become more popular since 2020 and video calls are often the communication channel of choice, but that doesn't mean your phone has become a white elephant. Whenever you get a phone call—it can be work-related or something more social—get up and walk around. It doesn't matter whether the call is less than a minute or 10 minutes long, move for the duration of the call.

Tip: Don't attempt a serious walk that will leave you breathy when taking more professional calls such as with clients. Keep the maximum effort phone walks for friends or colleagues.

Pacing

While pacing may not seem like much or an ideal way to walk, it will help you rack up your steps. Use a long hallway, large room, or even create your own home circuit from room to room. If you have a dedicated walking time every day, but can't get out of the house, this is a good option during your usual walk time.

Binge Walking

Binge-watching your favorite TV shows is something everybody has done. The problem is that you usually end up spending hours on the couch and your snack consumption goes through the roof. Swap being a couch potato for marching in place or walking on a treadmill while spending a few hours enjoying your guilty series-binging pleasure. You don't just have to binge-watch series to get moving in front of the TV. Is there a new movie you just have to watch? Step up the walking action for that hour and a half, or more, to help get to your step goal.

Podcast Pacing

Pacing around your home can become tedious and boring. Don't let the monotonous scenery put you off making your daily step goal. Listen to a podcast while you pace. Increase the benefit of podcast pacing by tuning into a podcast that offers you a chance at personal development for a physical, mental, and emotional workout all in one.

Tone Down Your Efficiency

Typically, chores are done at high speed to get them out of the way as quickly as possible. Being less efficient while doing household chores can help you increase your steps. Instead of trying to overload yourself carrying too many things from one room to the next—you know you're guilty of it—carry smaller amounts to increase walking back and forth. This can be extended to carrying groceries in from the car. Carry one bag in at a time instead of trying to heave several bags in at once.

Get Competitive

Friendly competition is a fantastic motivator to put in the extra effort to make as many steps as you can each day. A smartwatch is a perfect tool for connecting with friends and family by sharing your activity with them. Having a competitive nature spurs you on to try to beat your best friends or significant other, especially if there is some form of prize or reward involved.

Trampoline

Jumping up and down on a mini indoor trampoline might not seem like it has anything to do with walking, but it does actually count toward your step goal. Your body gets moving, your heart rate goes up, and your muscles get a workout. It's also kinder on your joints than running on a treadmill and more efficient.

Tip: Bungee trampolines are quieter and easier on your joints than spring trampolines.

Treadmill Desk

There are specially built standing desks that can accommodate an under-desk treadmill to enable you get more steps as you work. Other options include desk attachments for standard treadmills. It may take some getting used to at first and you won't be able to put in maximum effort, but a treadmill desk will keep you on the move instead of sitting on your butt for hours on end. You don't have to walk for the whole workday; alternate between a regular desk and a treadmill desk.

Additional Tips for Walking at Home

- Intentionally place items as far apart as possible. Put the printer on the other side of the room or in a different room entirely. If you have more than one bathroom, go to the one furthest away. Place the cups and coffee maker or kettle on opposite sides of the kitchen.
- Pace when you are trying to think of solutions to problems.
- Read emails on a tablet and pace around while reading them.
- Clear your mind when concentrating becomes more difficult by walking away from work for a few minutes or a set number of steps before coming back

and continuing.

CHANGING SPEED, INCLINES, AND RESISTANCE INDOORS

Walking indoors may seem to be limiting. Outdoor spaces offer the options of switching up the terrain, inclines, speeding up, and adding resistance to your walk. How can you enhance your indoor walks in a similar way to get the most benefit out of them?

Changing Speed

Treadmills offer the easiest and most effective option for walking faster indoors, but that isn't always possible if you don't have space or budget for a treadmill. If you have limited indoor space, try speeding up by taking shorter strides. If you are in a larger indoor space, such as a mall, try adding intervals to your walk by speeding up in open areas offering a straight line, and then slowing down in crowded spaces with lots of twists and turns.

Adding Inclines

There are no natural hills indoors, so changing your incline is going to take some ingenuity. Again, treadmills are the most obvious option for adding inclines to your walk, but not everybody has access to a treadmill. However, the obvious is not always the only option.

- Use the stairs in malls, at home, or at work instead of the escalator or elevator.
- Raise your knees higher when walking or marching in place.
- Use a stepper machine or a stepping block to simulate using stairs.

Ramp up the Resistance

Ankle, wrist, or hand weights can increase the resistance of your walk. You don't have to use weights only at home. Don't be shy about taking hand weights or wearing wrist or ankle weights out and about to the store or mall. Another way of increasing the resistance of your walk is to include some bodyweight exercises, such as walking lunges or shoulder presses with hand weights.

6

MAKE IT A LIFESTYLE: CREATING A HABIT OF WALKING

Walking, just like any other form of exercise, needs to become a habit for your regime to really take hold and stick. Think about other good daily habits you have, like brushing your teeth, for example. These good habits have become so ingrained in your daily life that they are almost automatic. To get the most out of walking, you need to make it a daily habit.

REPETITION CREATES ROUTINE

Any habit is formed through repetition. Repeating an action over and over again at the same time of day creates a routine. When you make walking a habit and part of your routine, it will become easy to stay on track with your walking program.

How Often to Walk

- Walk at least five times per week for weight loss.
- Walk at least three to four times per week for health benefits.
- Avoid skipping your walk for more than two consecutive days at a time.
- Walking training for distance or speed should be done six days per week with one day off. Alternate increased pace or distance days with slower or shorter distance days.

When to Walk

- Taking a walk first thing in the morning helps prevent procrastination, getting too busy or tired, and skipping your walk.
- Walking can be built into your work day by walking during breaks.
- Walking in the afternoon or evening may help you relax and clear your mind.

Build your walking schedule to suit your weight loss, health, and lifestyle needs so that it fits in with your regular routines. Commit to forming a walking habit, but be prepared for setbacks. There may be days when you can't walk at your scheduled time or at all. It is important to cut yourself some slack and then get right back on the horse the next day.

HABIT-FORMING MOTIVATION

Putting the effort into forming a new habit takes motivation. There are two types of motivation you can draw from when you are trying to create a walking habit; internal and external motivators.

External Motivation

External motivation comes from sources outside of yourself. These motivators often come from seeking acceptance, recognition, social pressure, and avoiding negativity from others. Some examples may be:

- Wanting to look a certain way because it's more socially acceptable.
- Losing weight to avoid negative comments.
- Entering and placing well in a walking event to impress others.

The problem with external motivation is that it often fails to keep you motivated in the long run. Making others happy doesn't necessarily make you happy. When your personal happiness is at stake, you are much more likely to form a long-lasting good habit.

Internal Motivation

Internal motivation comes from within yourself. It's the motivation from things you want to feel and achieve for yourself and not for others. Some examples may be:

- Reaching personal health goals.
- Alleviating health conditions through fitness and weight loss.
- Wanting to feel healthier and fitter.

Internal motivation does the trick every time because it's something you want for yourself. The trick is finding the internal motivation to get you walking and keep you walking. To discover what your internal motivation is, grab a pen and paper and jot down a list of the reasons you're starting a walking program. Once you've written down all those reasons, divide them into internal and external motivation categories.

Tip: If your internal motivation list is looking a little short, try researching the benefits of walking to give you more reasons to add to your list.

EASE INTO IT

An obstacle that we often put in our own paths when we want to form a new fitness habit is that we try to do too much, too quickly. When you overload yourself and find you can't meet those initial goals, your motivation takes a serious knock and you risk breaking the cycle of forming a walking habit.

When beginning any fitness routine, start out slowly and build yourself up to bigger, better things. Start out with a goal you think may even be too easy; see how your body responds, and gradually increase the step/distance/speed goal as you go along. Each time you increase any aspect of your walking, allow your body to get used to it for a few days. The first day may feel fine, but after a few consecutive days, you may be rethinking the idea to increase it again too soon because it seemed easy on day one.

BUILDING BLOCKS OF FORMING A HABIT

The author of The Power of Habit, Charles Duhigg, laid out the three repetitive components of forming a habit.

Cue: The habit trigger can be anything from a physical setting to a specific time of day. Find what prompts you to get walking.

Routine: Your walking routine consists of the things you do and think before, during, and after walking.

Reward: Your walking reward is the result you get from it. The result of your walking should align with your goals or the reason you're walking.

Create an action plan using your walking cue, what your walking routine is or will look like, and what the outcomes are or will be, to help make your intention of forming this habit stronger.

BUILDING MOMENTUM

If you are new to walking, you can imagine yourself as a ball lying on the ground at the top of a gentle slope. You're not going anywhere at the moment and it will take some effort to get moving, but once you're rolling down that slope, you build momentum and continuing to roll becomes much easier.

- Building momentum doesn't mean walking every single day. It means putting the effort in to walk on every single day you planned to walk.
- On planned walk days, try to at least start your walk. You can always stop if you really can't complete the whole walk. Even if you don't think you can do something, once you start, you are more likely to persevere to the end.
- Concerning breaking through resistance barriers to maintain your momentum, unless you really cannot walk or need a rest day, don't let a lack of motivation or listlessness talk you into skipping a walk.
- Don't skip too many consecutive walk days. Motivation can peter out quickly with each passing

day without walking.

BE COMPASSIONATE WITH YOURSELF

We are quick to beat ourselves up for not reaching goals or not walking on every planned walking day. Life can sometimes get in the way of our best intentions. Illness, injury, emergencies and various obstacles will come along. Being too hard on yourself when you don't do as well as you expect, or even fail, increases the risk of giving up completely. Why? Dwelling on what has just happened and beating yourself up over it keeps you stuck in that negative experience instead of looking to the future and what you're going to do next. Practice self-compassion by:

- Acknowledging and accepting that we all falter and sometimes fail; it's what makes us human.
- Avoiding harsh self-criticism.
- Not suppressing negative emotions or blowing them out of proportion; acknowledge disappointment, accept it, and let it go.
- Speaking to yourself kindly.

START ENJOYING WALKING

Nobody wants to do anything that isn't enjoyable. The enjoyment factor of an activity instantly increases the motivation needed to make it stick as a habit. To make your walks more enjoyable:

- Invest in comfortable—even fashionable—walking gear that makes you feel good.
- Switch up your route or take your walks in more enjoyable environments.
- Turn up the tunes, podcasts, or audiobooks.
- Walk with friends or join a walking group.
- Practice mindfulness or do some introspection while walking.
- Reward yourself for achieving your goals.

KEEP EXPECTATIONS IN CHECK

As we've said before in our goal-setting section, keep your expectations and goals realistic. If you set your sights too high over the short term, you're bound to be disappointed and may risk throwing in the towel. Disappointment isn't good when you're trying to build a new habit, so check out that goal-setting advice again to keep your expectations in check for forming a walking habit.

MAKE WALKING A NON-WORKOUT HABIT

Do you know about NEAT? Non-exercise activity thermogenesis is a really big name for small things you do every day that burn calories. Everything you do in your life that isn't planned exercise falls under NEAT. Okay, sleeping, eating, and breathing aren't NEAT, but everything else is. Walking, when not done as a planned exercise, contributes to your daily NEAT calorie burn.

Make walking a habit to get extra steps in and burn more calories by:

- Taking the stairs.
- Walking to nearby destinations instead of driving.
- Parking further from a building entrance rather than closer.
- Walking and talking to friends or colleagues instead of sitting down. You can even suggest walking meetings instead of sitting around a boardroom table.
- Taking your dates outdoors and walking instead of sitting across a table from each other.
- Using public transport instead of driving; you usually have to do a little walking to get to and from public transport.

Look for ways to incorporate walking into your life that don't leech time out of an already busy day. You are more likely to make walking a natural habit if it's part of something you already do and doesn't eat into your leisure time.

7

TRACKING, MONITORING, AND MEASURING YOUR RESULTS

Undertaking a walking program is a big step toward your health, fitness, and weight loss goals. Tracking your progress is part of staying motivated to keep going. Your motivation will vary from day to day; being able to look back and see how far you've come is a great pick-me-up when you're feeling less than enthusiastic about walking.

WHAT TO TRACK

- Steps taken: 10,000-step goal.
- Distance.
- Time: Work up to 150 minutes of brisk walking per week.
- Speed.

- Calories: Both for walking and your total daily calorie burn.

Many fitness tracking gadgets and apps will help record these figures for you, taking some of the work off your plate, but you still have to keep an eye on the numbers to monitor your progress.

How to Use Walking Data

Recorded data can help you identify patterns to improve and maximize your walking program.

- Is your activity level higher during the week or over weekends?
- Is your performance better when walking alone or with a friend?
- What time of day are you more likely to exercise?
- Are you reaching your daily or weekly goals?

Important note: Adjust or lower your goals if you aren't reaching them. When you can comfortably reach your target, raise them by smaller amounts to make them more achievable and maintain motivation.

Printable Walking Trackers

Having a printed tracking log for your progress and pinning it in a place where you can see it regularly could help keep you on track.

Important note: You can choose to record your pace or your speed. They may seem like the same thing, but they are not quite the same.

- The pace is the time taken to cover a unit of distance. For example, eight minutes per mile.
- Speed is the distance covered per unit of time. For example, walking at eight minutes per mile gives you a speed of 7.5 miles per hour.

You can record one or the other or both, depending on what your walking goals are. We've provided you with space to record both.

Notes about your walk could be anything you want to keep track of or remember. For example, perceived exertion, how you felt, etc.

Weekly Walking Log

\multicolumn{6}{c}{Weekly Walking Log Week ___ of walking program}						
Day-Date	Distance km/mi	Time	Pace/Speed	Steps	Notes	
Monday __/__/__						
Tuesday __/__/__						
Wednesday __/__/__						
Thursday __/__/__						
Friday __/__/__						
Saturday __/__/__						
Sunday __/__/__						
Weekly Totals						
Step goal increase:							
Progress made this week:							
Ideas for improvement/change:							

Daily Walking Journal

Daily Walking Journal Day:_____ Date: __/__/__					
Walk/Route	Distance km/mi	Time	Pace/Speed	Steps	Notes
Achievements					
Companions & effect on walking					
Observations					
New Goals					
Ideas					

ACTIVITY TRACKERS

Pedometers are out and activity or fitness trackers are in. Unlike pedometers, they count more than just your steps to give you a clearer overall picture of your progress.

Activity trackers differ by make and model, but some of the things many can track may include:

- What type of activity you're doing.
- The distance you've covered.
- Your heart rate.
- Calorie intake and calorie burn.
- Sleep patterns.
- Set alarms.
- Be used as a watch.

Activity tracker design varies greatly between brands and models, but most look like wristwatches and can be worn all the time. Modern activity trackers can be linked to other smart devices such as smartphones, computers, and tablets through apps and websites. These smart gadgets can even help set goals, provide cues to get moving if you've been sitting still for a while, and provide personal achievement awards to keep you motivated. Many fitness trackers can be linked to apps like Strava, where you can share your progress with friends, encouraging friendly competition.

Why Invest In an Activity Tracker

You can set short- and long-term goals on your activity tracker through a compatible app. Goals may include steps and activity time per week. By looking at the device, you can instantly see how many steps you have taken at any time in the day. The tracker will track your activity and reflect that data against your set goals. Once you reach a goal, you can set another one. A tracker will also serve as a reminder of what your goals are.

When you first start using an activity tracker, you can use the data to determine your average amount of daily activity to establish a baseline. Your baseline will give you a good idea of what kind of short- and long-term goals to set that are both realistic and achievable.

You can track your activity more accurately. Some activity trackers will record your activity on a weekly or even monthly basis. If your tracker doesn't have that feature, you can use the printable logs to monitor your progress or an app that records your activity on a weekly, monthly, and even yearly basis.

Making the Right Choice

Choosing the right activity tracker is a personal choice, based on the features you want and your budget.

- Price: Price will be the first and foremost deciding factor. The more features it has, the higher the price.

- Ease of use: More features can mean that they are more complicated to use, but most are relatively easy to use, once the tracker is set up.
- Features: How you intend to use a tracker and what data you want to record may determine the tracker you choose.
- Style: Various makes and models are available, some more fashionable than others. Depending on whether you are going to wear the tracker all the time, you may want one that looks more like a watch to complement various outfits.
- Additional: Whether you want to do water sports and how often you charge the tracker are considerations to take into account.
- Display: Lighting and how many features you want to see at the same time.
- Accuracy: Some trackers are more accurate than others.

How to Buy an Activity Tracker

The quality of the activity data your tracker collects can vary greatly from one brand to the next and one model to the next. Depending on the brand you choose, the algorithms not only collect, but also analyze the data, making the make just as important as the quality of the sensors in them.

Fitbit and Garmin often have higher-quality data collection and analysis than other emerging brands, making them more reliable for a better overall experience. They also offer better apps to track more data, improving motivation.

However, that doesn't mean you have to have the latest and greatest device. If you are looking for simple data to be recorded, you can opt for an emerging brand that isn't as pricey. Let's take a look at a rundown of the fitness tracker brands and models that have been voted the most popular in 2021 by the users, reviews, and testing.

Specs	Fitness Tracker				
Best for:	Fitness band for the average person	Fitness watch	Fitness band for the average person	Outdoor fitness watch	Budget
	Fitbit Charge 4	Garmin Vivosmart 4	Fitbit Inspire 2	Garmin Fenix 6	Xiaomi Mi Band 5
Compatibility	Android and iOS	Android and iOS	Android and iOS	Android and iOS	Android and iOS
Battery life	7 days	7 days	10 days	14 days	14 days
Heart rate monitor	Yes	Yes	Yes	Yes	Yes
Sleep monitor	Yes	Yes	Yes	Yes	Yes
Step tracker	Yes	Yes	Yes	Yes	Yes
Waterproof	Up to 50m	Up to 50m	Up to 5m	Up to 100m	Up to 50m
Smartphone notifications	Yes	Yes	Yes	Yes	Yes
GPS	Built-in	Connects to smartphone	Built-in	Built-in	Connects to smartphone
Companion app	Yes	Yes	Yes	Yes	Yes

WALKING APPS

Walking apps are another great way to track your walking fitness progress. They can be used in conjunction with other wearables such as fitness bands and watches. Walking apps are available on both Android and iOS smartphones, come in free and paid options, and come with a variety of features ranging from basic walking tracking to social features.

Basic tracking features may include:

- Steps.
- Distance.
- Speed.
- Calories burned.
- Activity level.
- Routes taken.

Social features may include sharing statistics, walking routes, and photos with other walkers.

Best Walking Apps

New apps are coming out all the time. Here's a rundown of the top picks for 2021.

MapMyWalk

Part of the MapMyFitness group of fitness apps, MapMy-Walk has been around for a while and is a firm favorite among fitness walkers.

- The app is available on Android and iOS.
- MapMyWalk is compatible with other wearables and apps such as smartwatches and fitness bands.
- Premium membership unlocks additional features.
- If you want to do more than walk, there are over 600 trackable activities to choose from.
- Walks can be uploaded and saved to be viewed both on the MapMyWalk website and mobile app.
- A map of the area is shown at the start of your walk.
- Walking progress is tracked on the map in real time.
- Route tracking allows exploring without getting lost.
- You can view routes other MapMyWalk users have taken to try out new routes.
- During your walk, statistics are displayed such as distance, time, speed, calories, and elevation.
- Speed is tracked using your phone's GPS.
- The mile-by-mile splits allow you to analyze your walking performance.
- Audio feedback is offered during your walk, letting you know your speed, distance, calories, etc. at intervals.

Argus by Azumio

The Argus app is an all-in-one fitness lifestyle app that does so much more than just track your walking. It's jam-packed with features to promote interaction with the app and a holistically healthy lifestyle.

- Argus is available on Android and iOS
- Upgrade to a premium subscription to unlock diet and fitness plans.
- Pedometer allows all-day step counting using your phone's motion sensor, including an hourly graph, steps, distance, time spent active, and calories.
- Workout statistics include distance, time, and route map.
- After a walking workout, steps, best and average pace, calories, distance, map, graphs, and average cadence can be viewed.
- Routes are tracked using your phone's GPS.
- The integrated heart rate app reads your heart rate by placing your index finger on the camera lens.
- The food diary includes a barcode scanner.
- Tap to track your water intake.
- There is a built-in sleep timer.
- Argus can be linked to a heart rate monitor band.

Walkmeter Walking and Hiking GPS by Abvio

The Walkmeter app is ideal for fitness walkers. It can help work on your distance and walking speed with features like intervals, splits, zones, etc.

- Walkmeter is available on Android, iOS, and Apple Watch.
- Upgrading to a paid subscription unlocks features such as cadence, steps, coaching, and treadmill.

- Your mobile phone's GPS is used to track distance.
- Stop and start your walk using Siri voice commands or your earphone remote.
- Walks are mapped out while walking.
- Statistics such as distance, speed, and time can be viewed while walking.
- Voice and audio capabilities provide feedback about your walk statistics. You can also hear replies to your walking workout from Twitter and Facebook as you go along.
- Pit yourself against your previous statistics or the stats of others on the same route.
- Walking workouts can be set up using tempo or repeating intervals.
- Training plans for distance walking are provided, including marathon, half-marathon, 10km, and 5km. You are also able to design your own training plan and sync it to your iPhone calendar.

Virtual Walk

- Virtual Walk is available on Android and iOS.
- Walk your way through renowned walking and hiking routes virtually on your mobile device.
- Use the app indoors or outdoors.
- At distance points, information and photographs about the sights and points of interest along your chosen route are provided.

- Virtual Walk routes include the Pyramids of Giza, Washington DC's mountains, the Appalachian Trail, the Grand Canyon, and many others.
- A medal is provided once you have completed a route.

Charity Miles

Make your steps count with the Charity Miles app by earning a donation to your charity of choice for every mile completed. Roughly 25 cents is donated for each mile walked or run and 10 cents per mile cycled.

Important note: Earning donations for charity may be subject to be capped periodically.

- The app offers minimal fitness tracking, but can be used at the same time as other apps so you can still track your fitness while walking for charity.
- Come together with friends or other walkers to form teams to raise money.
- Time and miles can be viewed while walking.
- After walking, a post to social media, Twitter or Facebook, is a must for sponsorship acceptance and the donation to be made.

Fitbit App Mobile Tracker

- No Fitbit fitness tracking wearable needed to make use of the Fitbit app.
- It is available on Android, iOS, and Windows mobile phones.
- Pedometer uses your phone's motion sensor to track all-day steps. Hourly graphs provide a visual representation of your statistics.
- Fun challenges and virtual adventure competitions add a competitive twist for motivation.
- The track exercise function allows you to record distance and speed when walking, running or hiking.
- Your phone's GPS tracks walking workouts.
- Voice prompts and audio updates are provided during your walk.
- You can view statistics such as time and average speed while walking.
- Swiping the screen shows you a map of your route progress.
- After a walk, you can view your route map, time, distance, speed, mile-by-mile splits, steps, and calories.

Endomondo

If you're looking for an app that's going to simulate being your personal trainer, Endomondo is your app.

- Exercise options include walking, fitness walking, hiking, and treadmill walking.
- Types of workouts include basic, route-based, and goal-targeted (time, distance, or calorie burn).
- Create your own route or follow routes others have taken.
- The app is available on Android, iOS, and Apple Watch.
- Users must upgrade the subscription to make use of a step counter.
- A premium subscription unlocks the step counter, heart rate zones, visual representations in graphs, training plans for runners, being able to compete against your own previous statistics, and interval training.
- Endomondo can be connected to other activity monitoring accounts, such as Fitbit.
- Your route map and walking statistics can be viewed while you walk.
- Audio feedback provides you with time, lap time, distance, other statistics, and even a pep talk.
- Outdoor activity tracking uses your phone's GPS.
- After your walk, you can view your route map, distance, time, average and maximum speed, minimum and maximum altitude, total elevation gain, hydration, calories, and total elevation loss.
- The app can be linked to a heart rate monitor.
- Connect with others using the app.

- Share your workouts on social media.

MotionX GPS

- The app is not available on Android. It is only available on iOS and Apple Watch.
- Outdoor activities are tracked, showing distance, speed, and time.
- Route maps of areas worldwide are available.
- Choose from 14 different types of maps, including road, satellite view, topographic, Bing and Google maps, and NOAA marine charts (experimental).
- Route maps can be stored for offline use, which is handy if you are walking or hiking in an area with bad or no reception.
- Live tracking is displayed on any type of map.
- You can view position, altitude, elevation gain and loss, speed, time, and gradient information.
- Up to 2,500 personal waypoints and 300 tracks can be saved to the app.
- Take geotagged photos during your walk to share on social media.
- You can be your own tour guide with Wikipedia integration.
- An interactive stopwatch and voice coaching are available.

PART II

8

HIGH-QUALITY NUTRITION AND HEALTHY FOODS TO SUPPORT YOUR WALKS

There's a reason they say that diet and exercise go hand-in-hand when it comes to both health and weight loss. Some people operate under the misconception that they can maintain an unhealthy diet, but if they just add a ton of exercise, the weight will still come off and they will improve their health. This is, in fact, not true at all. For holistic health and effective, sustainable weight loss, exercise only contributes about 15 percent to the effect; the remaining 85 percent is made up by diet.

Proper diet and nutrition aren't just necessary to help you lose weight and get healthy. What you eat fuels your walking. If you aren't topping the tank up with quality fuel, your body isn't going to perform as well. You may even end up falling short of your goals simply because your body isn't getting what it needs to function properly.

Important note: Good nutrition can help prevent, reverse, or manage a variety of health conditions, such as cardiovascular disease and diabetes. Poor nutrition can have the opposite effect, making health conditions worse or even making you more susceptible to developing them.

CALORIES VERSUS NUTRITION

When the topic of losing weight comes up, your first thought may be severe portion restrictions and carefully counting each and every calorie. The truth is, that's not how weight loss really works. It may show small yields in the short term, but many people who crash diet end up piling the weight back on once they stop dieting. There are a few reasons why nutrition is king when it comes to healthy weight loss, so get ready to ditch the calorie-counting obsession.

Calorie Deficit Fallacy

The most commonly observed practice for weight loss is to create a calorie deficit. The principle says that, if you consume fewer calories per day than you expend, your body will have to dig into its fat stores to make up the rest of what it needs. The problem with this theory, as modern medical science is starting to suggest, is that it doesn't necessarily work. Your body is built to survive and when it senses a calorie deficit, it perceives that deficit as famine. Instead of letting you burn your way through those calories fast and furiously, it's going to do whatever it can to hold on to as much of your body fat for as long as possible.

The result of a calorie deficit may be that your metabolism slows down by as much as 30 percent. Let that sink in. If you need to take in 1,800 calories per day to maintain your weight, reducing that by 500 calories per day should result in a loss of approximately one pound per week. If your metabolism slows down by 30 percent, you would only need 1,260 calories per day. Here's the math: 1,800 − 500 = 1,300. Effectively, what this would mean is that you would maintain weight instead of losing it.

One of the biggest problems with today's modern Western diet is that it includes too many empty calories and not enough proper nutrition. Slimming down doesn't need a drastic calorie slash, but it does need high-quality nutrition. Why? Weight loss starts with the individual cells in your body.

For your body to efficiently burn fat stores, your body's cells must be in tip-top shape. Without proper nutrition, your cells won't be as healthy as they could be. Cellular repair will also suffer, resulting in slower repair and regeneration of unhealthy cells. Providing your cells with the proper nutrition increases their fat-burning power. Proper nutrition may also improve your sleep. The more sleep you get and the better the quality of your sleep, the more efficiently your body can repair and regenerate cells.

INSULIN AND WEIGHT GAIN

Insulin is the villain in your weight loss story. To understand how changing your diet can help you lose weight without having to drastically cut your calories, you need to know how insulin works and why it can be such a weight loss enemy.

- The food you eat is broken down during digestion.
- Carbohydrates are broken down into the simplest sugars and absorbed into your bloodstream.
- When your blood sugar level rises, your pancreas releases insulin.
- Insulin removes the sugar from your blood, transporting it to individual cells where it's used for fuel.
- When your cells have been refueled, excess sugar is turned into glycogen and stored in your muscles as quick-access reserves.
- Once those glycogen stores are full, the leftover sugar is turned into fat and stored.

This process happens every time you eat. Every time your blood sugar spikes, insulin is released. The problem with the typical Western diet is that it's laden with carbohydrates, causing big blood sugar spikes and lots of excess sugar. Over time, consistently consuming too many carbohydrates renders your insulin less effective, leading to insulin resistance where your body is being constantly flooded with insulin to try to control blood sugar levels. More and more fat is stored and you become constantly hungry because the blood sugar is being removed as quickly as you can replace it. It becomes a vicious cycle. Left unchecked, insulin resistance can lead to diabetes, resulting in constantly high blood sugar levels because insulin stops working for your body.

Reducing Carbs

To counteract the weight-gain effect insulin has on your body, you need to control the number of carbohydrates you eat as well as the quality of those carbs.

- Reduce refined and processed sugars. These sugars are easy to break down quickly, causing blood sugar spikes. They are found in everyday food items you probably didn't realize contained added sugar. Some of the culprits include corn sweetener, fructose, glucose, high-fructose sweetener, hydrolyzed starch, invert sugar, and sucralose.
- Reduce refined grains such as white flour, white rice, baked goods, etc. Opt for whole-grain bread, cereals, pasta, and other whole-grain foods.
- Eat protein in moderation as a good source of amino acids. Protein helps keep you feeling fuller longer.
- Choose whole, fresh foods or foods that have been minimally processed instead of highly refined and processed foods found in packages, cans, and bottles.

Whole foods make you feel fuller quicker, making it harder to overeat. They are also naturally lower in calories, while being denser in nutrition.

PORTION CONTROL

Even foods labeled as healthy can lead to unintentional difficulties in weight loss or even gaining weight if you do not control your portion sizes. Knowing the right portion sizes can help you determine what's on your plate:

- Calories.
- Carbs.
- Fats.
- Protein.
- Sodium.

When you know what's on your plate, you can eat with peace of mind, knowing that the amount is just right.

Serving Size and Portion Size

Don't get serving size and portion size confused.

- Serving size: The amount of a specific type of food normally eaten in a single sitting as determined by the Food and Drug Administration (FDA).
- Portion size: How much of a particular food you actually eat.

Your dished portion is bigger than a serving size, misleading you into believing you are eating fewer calories than you really are. For example, a heaped tablespoon of peanut butter could contain twice the amount of calories as a properly measured tablespoon.

Correctly calculating portion size based on your personal daily caloric and carb intake needs is a vital tool for achieving weight loss success. You are a unique person; the correct portion for someone else may not be right for you. Your portions should be based on what you need to eat per day to be healthy, keep your body fueled, and not leave you feeling deprived.

Portion Control Tips

- Specifically designed portion control dishes, glasses, and spoons will help you shift away from estimating and toward properly measuring food according to what you actually need to be eating.
- A food scale can help you accurately measure the amount of food you want to eat by weight, whether it's dry weight or fluid weight.
- Use smaller plates, bowls, and glasses to encourage you to eat smaller portions. A portion appears bigger on a smaller plate while you could be fooled into thinking that it's smaller than it really is by dishing it up on a larger plate with plenty of open space all around.

- Be wary of condiments and measure them out carefully. Condiments could have hidden sugar and carbs in them so don't treat them as *free* additions to your diet.

WATER FOR WEIGHT LOSS

Considering that the majority of your body is made up of water, it stands to reason that water plays a vital role in a variety of bodily functions that influence weight loss. These functions range from how well your muscles perform to the digestion of food. The better your body works, the better your weight loss results will be. So, why wouldn't you want to make sure that you drink enough water?

Weight Loss Benefits

There are six suggested reasons why drinking enough water could aid you on your weight loss journey.

Water Is Vital For Walking

Walking is a gentle exercise, but it's still exercising. Every part of your body that is working while walking—lungs, muscles, joints, organs, and connective tissues—rely on water to move and function. If you don't drink enough water, you could become dehydrated and suffer complications such as fatigue and muscle cramps which could ruin your workout.

Appetite Suppressant

Water serves as a natural appetite suppressant. Have you ever been told to drink a glass of water when you complained about being hungry, despite having eaten only a short while before? There's logic in that suggestion. Being thirsty can mimic the same feeling as hunger, confusing your brain as to whether you need to eat or drink something. By reaching for a glass of water before you decide to have a snack, you could quench your thirst masquerading as hunger, and prevent yourself from snacking when you're not really hungry at all.

Drinking water before or during a meal helps to take up space in your stomach. This tricks you into feeling fuller faster and helps you eat less in a single sitting.

Burning Calories

It's suggested that drinking water that is either cold or room temperature may actually slightly increase the number of calories your body burns for a period after drinking it. Drinking cold water can have an additional calorie-burning effect. Drinking cold water lowers your core temperature, prompting your body to expend more energy to heat itself up again and to warm the water for digestion.

Water Helps Burn Fat

Water is a vital component in the metabolic equation when burning carbs or fat for fuel. Without enough water, you cannot burn your stored fat for fuel. Nor can you properly burn off the energy you just took in from a meal. If you want to burn fat, ditch the other beverages and reach for water instead.

Lowering Liquid Calories

Water is completely calorie-free. It's natural, it's healthy, and it can help you stop drinking your calories. It's easy to overlook the calories in a cup of coffee, a can of soda, or a bottle of energy drink. All too often, we reach for non-water forms of hydration that make the calories stack up and don't provide us with the proper hydration our bodies are asking for. Filling up on water means you're less likely to fill up on empty calories.

Waste Elimination

A properly hydrated body can eliminate waste and toxins while a dehydrated body can't do it as efficiently. If your body can't flush the toxins out, they hang around and have a negative effect on your body's cells. Remember what we said about your body needing to function properly and your cells needing to be healthy for optimal weight loss progress? Well, having toxins in your body doesn't keep your cells healthy which may impede your progress. If that wasn't bad enough, these same toxins can lead to bloating, making your midsection bigger than it really is.

9

TRACKING AND MONITORING YOUR WEIGHT LOSS

Tracking your weight loss progress can be a big motivator to help you stick to your walking program and keep pushing yourself to meet non-weight loss walking goals. Aside from keeping tabs on your physical weight loss, it is also important to keep track of your daily food intake. It's not all about calories when your aim is healthy, safe weight loss and overall improved health.

Important note: Losing weight too quickly can be dangerous to your health. A healthy, safe weight loss goal is between one and two pounds per week. It can be tempting to try to shed the weight faster, but slower, healthier weight loss is the key to not only losing weight, but keeping it off in the long term.

TRACK YOUR FOOD

Tracking your food intake doesn't have to be about weighing food and counting every calorie. There are a few simple tricks that can help you keep an eye on what you eat without focusing on a small part of the bigger picture.

FOOD JOURNALING

Keeping a food journal is an effective way to help you make better food choices. How? It's simple; you give more thought to what you are choosing to eat when you have to keep a record by writing it down. Keeping a food journal will help you identify your eating habits and patterns so that you can make changes to adopt a healthier diet.

Mobile App Food Journaling

YouAte is a free mobile app, available on Android and iOS, that will help you log what you eat without having to carry a physical journal and pen around. In fact, using this app is so easy that you don't have to make notes about your meals at all. All you do is take a photograph of your meal and mark it as either "on-path" or "off-path." That's it. You also have the power to decide what on- and off-path means to you, personally, instead of trying to rate your food choice by standards that may not be in line with your goals. This nifty app will provide you with feedback on what percentage of your meals were on or off the path at the end of each week.

There are additional features when logging meals that can give you greater insight into your food patterns. Some simple questions can be answered when you log a meal:

- Why did you eat? Answer options include "It was time," "Cravings," and "Hungry."
- Who did you eat with? Answer options include friends, family, social, etc.
- How was it? Explain how the food was; was it good, bad, average, etc.?
- Where did you eat? Answer options include "At a table," "Car," "TV," and even "Work desk," and more.
- How was it made? Was it home cooked, convenience meal, fast food, etc.?
- How did it make you feel? Did you feel satisfied, guilty, still hungry, etc.?

Traditional Food Journaling

If using an app just isn't your thing, keep it old-school by journaling your food in a physical journal or on a mobile device in a more traditional way.

Rules to follow when using a food journal:

- Write down absolutely everything, even if you take a bite of a friend's meal.
- Write it down at the moment, and don't wait because you might forget.

- Write down specifics; don't use blanket terms. If you ate fish sticks, note fish sticks and not just fish.
- Estimate how much food you are eating. Estimations can range from physical sizes, such as inches, to measurements like teaspoons and cups. A handy tip is that a portion of cooked meat weighing three ounces is roughly the size of a deck of cards.

When writing down your food intake, remember to include the following:

- How much of it you ate, estimated serving size, or the number of individual items. For example, ½ cup of rice or three cookies.
- What you ate, and the type of food or drink you consumed. Remember to be specific and not to disregard additional toppings, sauces, or additions such as sugar, butter, and mustard.
- The time of day you eat or drink anything.
- Where you eat or drink it. Again, be specific. Don't just note that you were at home; note the room you were in and if you were sitting at a table or on the sofa, etc.
- Who you ate with, such as alone, with friends, family, coworkers, etc.
- What you were doing when you ate it, such as driving, working, sitting in front of the TV, etc.

- How you felt when you ate it. How you feel can influence when you eat and what you eat.

For example:

How much	What	Time	Where	Who with	Activity	Mood
1 x 2 oz. bag	BBQ-flavored (brand name) chips	2:00 p.m.	Car	Alone	Driving	Stressed

A journal entry like this would indicate that you were indulging in unhealthy snack food alone in your car while driving. You were feeling stressed. Now ask yourself, were you eating that out of hunger, or were you stress-eating? A food journal provides insight into your eating patterns in an effective, visible way.

Important note: For a food journal to be successful, you must be 100 percent honest in writing down absolutely everything and a portion estimation that is as close to accurate as possible.

HEALTHY FOOD CHOICE APPS

Shopwell: Free

- Scan grocery store items for information in it.
- Find out the health rating, how to use it, similar alternatives, etc.

- This app is useful for ensuring you stick to a specific diet, such as gluten-free.

Eating Well: Free

- Provides lots of tasty, healthy recipes.
- Recipes are suggested based on the food you want to eat and health/weight loss goals.
- Nutritional value per serving is provided with recipes.

Fooducate: Free

- Educate yourself on the value of quality calories, not quantity.
- Track meals and hunger patterns.
- Get recipe ideas.
- Track sleeping patterns.

Rise: Variable

- Subscription is required for some services offered.
- Team up with a nutritionist.
- Create a personalized diet plan.
- Photograph and share your meals for tips.
- Get support from your coach when you need help.

The Blender Girl: Paid

- Available on iOS.
- Homemade smoothie recipes are provided based on your mood and how you want your smoothie to make you feel.
- Draw up a smoothie grocery list to remember what goes into your smoothies.

Harvest: Paid

The app provides suggestions for fresh, in-season produce and how to use it.

Nom Nom Paleo: Paid

- Get help following the paleo diet with recipes, ingredient shortcuts, and tips.
- Create a paleo-friendly shopping list to avoid confusion in the store.

TRACK YOUR WEIGHT LOSS

You are undertaking a life-changing new walking-for-weight-loss program. It is crucial that you keep track of your weight loss progress. Tracking your weight loss is incredibly motivational. It can help keep you going when you lack motivation, feel like you aren't making progress, or lose sight of how far you've come.

The problem with tracking weight loss is that it's often done using a traditional bathroom scale and you can become obsessed with and discouraged by the number on the scale. If the scale isn't playing ball and the number isn't coming down, you aren't necessarily hitting a weight loss plateau.

Bathroom scales are also known as bodyweight scales. They measure everything from body fat to muscle and water weight. They don't discriminate. If the number goes up, it can't tell you what you've gained. If the number goes down, it can't tell you whether your loss is from fat or something else.

Body Weight Fluctuations

Your body weight will fluctuate all the time, based on a variety of contributing factors. These factors are constantly changing, causing your weight to fluctuate without reflecting that you've actually lost or gained body fat.

- Water weight: Depending on how hydrated you are, how much salt you've eaten, or whether your hormones are fluctuating can cause your body to hold on to extra water. This water retention is reflected on the scale.
- Muscle weight: Muscle is denser than fat, weighing more. Building muscle through exercise may make the number of the scale go up while your physical size goes down.

- Food weight: The number on the scale will be higher after eating because you've added something to your body that will be digested, used for energy, and then eliminated.

Important note: If you know your body fat percentage, using a bodyweight scale gives you a more accurate picture of what is happening to your body. Using a scale alone may not be effective and could ultimately be detrimental to your motivation.

Tracking Body Fat

Think about a bodybuilder. Using a standard height-weight calculation such as body mass index (BMI), his result will tell him that he is overweight, despite having a very low body fat percentage. Muscle is dense and heavy; the more of it you have, the higher the number on the scale. Tracking your body fat percentage can be done in several ways.

- Bioelectrical impedance scales: Scales using a low-level electrical current to determine your lean mass combined with your total body weight, height, age, and gender to estimate body fat percentage.
- Calipers: Skinfold calipers measure how thick the layer of fat under the skin is in several spots on the body to estimate fat percentage.
- Online calculators: Possibly the least accurate and most basic form of estimating body fat percentage.

Consistency Is Key

Whether you are measuring your body fat percentage or your total body weight, remaining consistent is important.

Measure on the same day per week, at the same time of day, using the same device or having the same person measure you. Your weight will fluctuate at different times of the day and your body measurements will go up and down because of things like bloat after eating or drinking. Different scales will vary in their results even at the same time of day. Different people will measure you slightly differently, providing varying results.

Keep track of your measurements in a journal or on a calendar; it's a great way to hold yourself accountable.

Avoid measuring your progress too often, because change happens gradually and your body fluctuates from one day to the next. Expecting to see weight loss, but only seeing the same number or the numbers going up slightly, can be discouraging.

Tip: Weigh or measure yourself first thing in the morning. That is when you will be at your lowest weight and your body is unaffected by bloat that occurs while food is digesting.

Measuring Your Body

If the scale is discouraging and the body fat percentage is daunting to figure out, track your weight loss progress by measuring your body. Even if building muscle is duping the scale into telling you that you're not making progress, smaller measurements mean less fat.

Taking measurements in different areas helps you determine where you store most of your body fat and assures you that you are losing fat even if it's not happening as quickly in the areas you want to target.

Measuring your body naked is ideal, as there is no fabric to get in the way of accurate measurements. If you are clothed, make sure your clothing is skin-tight for the least amount of interference.

- Bust: Measure around your chest in line with your nipples.
- Calves: Measure around the biggest part of each calf.
- Chest: Measure around your chest, just under your bust or pectoral muscles.
- Forearm: Measure around the biggest part of your forearm below the elbow.
- Hips: Measure around the widest part of your hips.
- Thighs: Measure around the biggest section of each thigh.
- Upper arm: Measure around the biggest part of each upper arm above the elbow.
- Waist: Measure ½-inch above your belly button or around the smallest part of your waist.

Clothing and Photographs

You can judge your progress by feeling how your clothes fit. Choose an outfit that is tight-fitting. Put it on once a month to feel the difference as the clothes become looser with weight loss.

Try taking photographs of yourself in something fitted, such as underwear or a swimsuit. Try to take photographs from a few angles, such as front, back, and from the side. Repeat this process once a month to notice changes you may not be seeing because your eyes adjust as you lose weight. You may be surprised at the change; you could be so focused on your *problem* areas that you don't see changes elsewhere.

Weight Loss and Fitness Progress Chart

Below is a chart to help you keep track of your weight loss and fitness gains. If you don't know your body fat percentage, you can leave that one out.

Important note: Your resting heart rate (RHR) is a good reflection of increasing your fitness. The fitter you get, the lower your resting heart rate should be. Measure the number of beats per minute first thing in the morning or after at least four hours of resting after vigorous activity and several hours after eating:

Measurements	Date: __/__/__	Date: __/__/__	Date: __/__/__	Date: __/__/__	Date: __/__/__
Weight					
Body Fat					
RHR					
Bust					
Calves					
Chest					
Forearm					
Hips					
Thighs					
Upper Arm					
Waist					
Notes					

CONCLUSION

Walking is the way to a healthier, happier life. It's simple, it's accessible, and it works. Overlooking walking as a fantastic form of exercise to help you lose weight is a mistake that many people make, but not you—not anymore. You've made your way through our book and we've told you everything you need to know about walking to turn it into a lifestyle that will transform your health and fitness.

We've provided you with compelling information about the numerous health benefits you can take advantage of by simply getting up and walking. We've shared with you the knowledge of the various different types of walking, how to prepare, and how to get started. We've sold you on the practicality of walking, why it's effective, and why anybody can do it.

CONCLUSION

We have also provided you with a comprehensive seven-week beginner walking program to get you started and we've told you how to customize it to fit your personal needs and goals. We've even mentioned the importance of diet in weight loss and health, providing you with tips on how to improve your eating habits to help you reach your weight loss goals.

Walking is not just medicine; it's food for your body, mind, and spirit. It gives you a new lease on life as well as a new perspective on the world. The best part is that it is so simple that you could start right this minute.

So, the only question that remains is this: Now you have all the tools and resources you need, what are you waiting for?

Please leave a review on Amazon if you enjoyed the book.

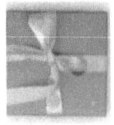 # A Free Bonus To Our Readers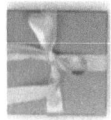

To get you started on your walking journey, we have created:

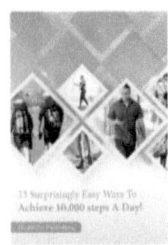 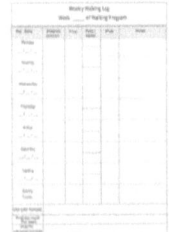 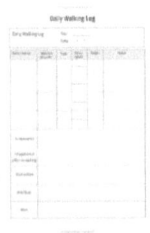 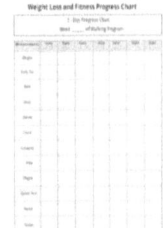

Free Bonus #1
23 Easy Ways To Achieve 10,000 Steps A Day

Free Bonus #2
A Weekly Walking Log

Free Bonus #3
A Daily Walking Log

Free Bonus #4
A Weight Loss and Fitness Progress Chart

With 23 Easy Ways to Achieve 10,000 Steps A Day, you get

- 10 health benefits of walking
- 9 risks associated with a sedentary lifestyle
- 23 different ways to achieve 10,000 steps each day

A Weekly Walking Log to record distance, time, speed/pace, steps and notes.

A Daily Walking Log to record walk/route, distance, time, pace/speed and notes.

A Weight Loss and Fitness Progress Chart to record weight, body fat, bust, hips, etc

To get your free bonuses, please click on the link or scan the QR code below and let us know the email address to send it to.

https://healthfitpublishing.com/bonus/wtwl/

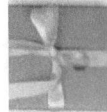 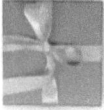

REFERENCES

"Computer vision syndrome. " by Wikipedia is licensed under CC BY-SA 4.0

"Sedentary lifestyle" by Wikipedia is licensed under CC BY-SA 4.0

4 reasons why walking outside benefits the brain. (2020, June 19). Advanced Neurotherapy. https://www.advancedneurotherapy.com/blog/2015/09/10/walking-outside-brain

7 ways to make everyday walking into a daily habit. (2019, January 21). The Pacer Blog. https://blog.mypacer.com/2019/01/21/7-ways-to-make-walking-into-your-everyday-habit/

REFERENCES

Alexas_Fotos. (2018, January 24). *The eleventh hour time to think disaster.* Pixabay. https://pixabay.com/photos/the-eleventh-hour-time-to-rethink-3101625/

Altmann, G. (2016, March 23). *Board step each other following in a row.* Pixabay. https://pixabay.com/illustrations/board-step-each-other-following-1273117/

Altmann, G. (2017, June 23). *Board school self confidence believe self-worth.* Pixabay. https://pixabay.com/photos/board-school-self-confidence-2433978/

Beginner's guide to Nordic pole walking. (2020, March 4). American Nordic Walking Association.

https://www.americannordicwalking.com/blog/2017/3/4/eo4yagte05ql8orxo5vnti12ze0d3n

Bjarnadottir, A. (2018, May 31). *The beginner's guide to the 5:2 diet.* Healthline. https://www.healthline.com/nutrition/the-5-2-diet-guide

Boone, T. (2007, December 4). *Benefits of walking.* How Stuff Works. https://health.howstuffworks.com/wellness/diet-fitness/exercise/benefits-of-walking.htm

Boyers, L. (3030, June 37). *How to reach your daily step golas when working from home.* Health And Wellness. https://www.cnet.com/health/how-to-reach-your-daily-step-goals-when-working-from-home/

REFERENCES

Breen, D. (2015, December 9). *Vegetables fruit food ingredients harvest produce*. Pixabay. https://pixabay.com/photos/vegetables-fruits-food-ingredients-1085063/

Brown, J. (2007, August 6). *The stroller workout*. Parents. https://www.parents.com/baby/health/lose-baby-weight/use-your-wheels-stroll-off-the-pounds/

Buissinne, S. (2015, June 1). *Printer desk office fax scanner home office*. Pixabay. https://pixabay.com/photos/printer-desk-office-fax-scanner-790396/

Bumgardner, W. (2019, June 24). *How to start walking for weight loss*. Verywell Fit. https://www.verywellfit.com/how-to-walk-for-beginners-3432464

Bumgardner, W. (2020, December 8). *The 8 best free walking apps for fitness walkers of 2021*. Verywell Fit. https://www.verywellfit.com/best-walking-apps-3434995

Bumgardner, W. (2020, January 22). *Starting a schedule to build your walking habit*. Verywell Fit. https://www.verywellfit.com/setting-a-walking-schedule-to-build-your-walking-habit-3435067

Bumgardner, W. (2020, November 20). *6 best ways to take your walking indoors*. Verywell Fit. https://www.verywellfit.com/best-ways-to-take-your-walking-indoors-3436836

Bumgardner, W. (2020, November 29). *Tracking your walks*. Verywell Fit. https://www.verywellfit.com/tracking-your-walks-3432825

REFERENCES

Bumgardner, W. (2021, March 15). *The 11 best indoor walking videos of 2021*. Verywell Fit. https://www.verywellfit.com/best-indoor-walking-videos-3435857

Burrell, J. (2021, March 29). What is geocaching? Verywell Family. https://www.verywellfamily.com/whats-inside-a-geocache-box-3570580

Carter, E. (2018, July 31). *The benefits of adding cross training to your exercise routine*. Michigan State University MSU Extension. https://www.canr.msu.edu/news/the_benefits_of_adding_cross_training_to_your_exercise_routine

Chertoff, J. (2018, November 8). *What are the benefits of walking?* Healthline. https://www.healthline.com/health/benefits-of-walking

Chhabra, A. (2020, May 4). *Types of walking for exercise*. The Institute For Weight Management. https://mdslim.com/wild-walks-different-types-of-walking-for-exercise/

Co-authored by Wikihow Staff. (2020, April 3). *How to do Nordic walking*. Wikihow. https://www.wikihow.com/Do-Nordic-Walking

Cordier, A. (2018, February 9). *5 reasons why warm up exercises are important*. Fit Athletic. https://fitathletic.com/5-reasons-warm-exercises-important/

Crady, M. (n.d.). *Pranayama for pedestrians*. Yoga International. https://yogainternational.com/article/view/pranayama-for-pedestrians

REFERENCES

de Cabo, R., & Mattson, M. P. (2019). Effects of Intermittent Fasting on Health, Aging, and Disease. *New England Journal of Medicine, 381*(26), 2541–2551. https://doi.org/10.1056/nejmra1905136

Dolson, L. (2020, December 16). *Non-exercise activity thermogenesis (NEAT) and health.* Verywell Fit. https://www.verywellfit.com/neat-non-exercise-activity-thermogenesis-2241984

Dreyer, D. (2011, August 3). *Build your core with chi walking.* Active. https://www.active.com/fitness/articles/build-your-core-with-chi-walking?page=2

Durward, L. (2017, July 20). *Workout Vaughan fitness squat barbell weights.* Pixabay. https://pixabay.com/photos/workout-vaughan-fitness-squat-2523087/

Enlarged heart. (2017). Mayo Clinic. https://www.mayoclinic.org/diseases-conditions/enlarged-heart/symptoms-causes/syc-20355436

Erofit & Associates. (2019, April 9). *How to race walk like an Olympian.* Verywell Fit. https://www.verywellfit.com/how-to-racewalk-p2-3436286

Exercise | meaning in the Cambridge English Dictionary. (2019). Cambridge Dictionary. https://dictionary.cambridge.org/dictionary/english/exercise

Exercise and your arteries. (2019, June 21). Harvard Health Publishing Harvard Medical School.https://www.health.

REFERENCES

harvard.edu/heart-health/exercise-and-your-arteries

Exercise: Starting a walking program. (n.d.). University Health Services UC Berkeley. https://uhs.berkeley.edu/health-topics/exercise-starting-walking-program

Family Doctor.org Editorial Staff. (2018, April 27). *Nutrition: Keeping a food diary.* Family Doctor.Org. https://familydoctor.org/nutrition-keeping-a-food-diary/

Fratti, K. (2017, August 10). *7 apps that can help you eat healthier without getting hung up on counting calories.* Hello Giggles. https://hellogiggles.com/lifestyle/health-fitness/7-apps-that-can-help-you-eat-healthier-without-getting-hung-up-on-counting-calories/

Free-Photos. (2016, August 21). *Coffee write planner journal hands table notebook.* Pixabay. https://pixabay.com/photos/coffee-write-planner-journal-hands-1246511/

Free-Photos. (2016, August 29). *Food fig fresh healthy vegetarian sandwich.* Pixabay. https://pixabay.com/photos/food-fig-fresh-healthy-vegetarian-1246640/

Freudenrich, C. (2000, October 27). *How fat cells work.* How Stuff Works. https://science.howstuffworks.com/life/cellular-microscopic/fat-cell2.htm

Fung J. (2021). Weight loss solution (step by step) | Jason Fung in *YouTube.* https://www.youtube.com/watch?v=OgmFEb0b0TI

REFERENCES

Get in the right mindset to exercise regularly. (2016, May 17). Psychcentral. https://psychcentral.com/lib/get-in-the-right-mindset-to-exercise-regularly#1

Getting started: A 6-week beginner walking program to get healthy. (2019, March 19). The Pacer Blog. https://blog.mypacer.com/2019/03/12/getting-started-a-beginner-walking-program-to-get-healthy/

Gunnars, K. (2020, April 20). *Intermittent fasting 101 – The ultimate beginner's guide.* Healthline. https://www.healthline.com/nutrition/intermittent-fasting-guide

Gunnars, K. (2020, January 1). *6 popular ways to do intermittent fasting.* Healthline. https://www.healthline.com/nutrition/6-ways-to-do-intermittent-fasting

How much physical activity do adults need? (2020, October 7). Centers for Disease Control & Prevention.

https://www.cdc.gov/physicalactivity/basics/adults/index.htm

Huizen, J. (2018, June 28). *Can water help you lose weight?* Medical News Today. https://www.medicalnewstoday.com/articles/322296

ID 5598375. (2018, April 22). *Sports Nordic walking woman girlfriends hike.* Pixabay. https://pixabay.com/photos/sport-nordic-walking-woman-3340697/

REFERENCES

Imeedy. (2015, May 7). *Road shoes walking sports run Taobao Mall.* Pixabay. https://pixabay.com/photos/road-shoes-walking-sports-run-749528/

It's time to learn about fasting. (2020, August 17). The Fasting Method. https://blog.thefastingmethod.com/the-science-of-intermittent-fasting/

Jarmoluk, M. (2015, August 26). *Stairs shopping mall shop shopping Kielce Crown.* Pixabay. https://pixabay.com/photos/stairs-shopping-mall-shop-shopping-906720/

Kandola, A. (2018, August 29). *What are the consequences of a sedentary lifestyle?* Medical News Today. https://www.medicalnewstoday.com/articles/322910

Kerckx, B. (2015, June 19). *Stretching sports jogger people legs.* Pixabay. https://pixabay.com/photos/stretching-sports-jogger-people-814227/

Kosecki, D. (2017, March 15). *The 5-minute stretching routine that will keep you walking strong.* Fitbit. https://uhs.berkeley.edu/health-topics/exercise-starting-walking-program

Kwan, N. (2011, November 3). *Yoga poses for walkers.* Prevention. https://www.prevention.com/fitness/fitness-tips/a20478110/yoga-positions-to-improve-walking-workouts/

Lashkari, C. (2016, October 9. *Where did 10,000 steps a day come from?* News Medical. https://www.news-medical.net/health/Where-did-10000-steps-a-day-come-from.aspx

Latona, V. (2019, May 29). *How to make that daily walk happen.* AARP. https://www.aarp.org/health/healthy-living/info-2019/making-walking-a-habit.html

Lindsay, M. (2018, November 3). *7 variations of walking that torch calories.* My Fitness Pal. https://blog.myfitnesspal.com/7-variations-of-walking-that-torch-calories/

Lindsay, M. (2019, July 25). *6 tips for walking with a baby stroller.* My Fitness Pal. https://blog.myfitnesspal.com/6-tips-for-walking-with-a-baby-stroller/

Lindsay, M. (2020, July 21). *10 common walking problems, solved.* My Fitness Pal. https://blog.myfitnesspal.com/common-walking-problems-solved/

Link, R. (2018, September 4). *16/8 intermittent fasting: A beginner's guide.* Healthline. https://www.healthline.com/nutrition/16-8-intermittent-fasting

Ludlum, K. (n.d.). *Stretching basics for walking.* Arthritis Foundation. https://www.arthritis.org/health-wellness/healthy-living/physical-activity/walking/stretching-basics-for-walking

Malacoff, J. (2020, January 17). *5 ways walkers van strengthen their arms.* My Fitness Pal. https://blog.myfitnesspal.com/5-ways-walkers-can-strengthen-their-arms/

REFERENCES

Mansour, S. (2020, May 6). *5 ways to supersize your walk.* CNN. https://edition.cnn.com/2020/05/06/health/exercise-fitness-walking-workout-quarantine-coronavirus-wellness/index.html

Martinac, P. (2019, July 8). *How eat-stop-eat works.* Livestrong. https://www.livestrong.com/article/438695-how-eat-stop-eat-works/

Maslakovic, M. (2020, September 26). Best fitness trackers and health gadgets for 2021. Gadgets & Wearables. https://gadgetsandwearables.com/2020/09/26/best-fitness-trackers-2020/?gclid=EAIaIQobChMI2ryusZeH8AIVjMLtCh1lfwNrEAAYAiAAEgKncvD_BwE

Mayo Clinic Staff. (n.d.). *Walking shoes: Features and fit that keep you moving.* Mayo Clinic. https://www.mayoclinic.org/healthy-lifestyle/fitness/in-depth/walking/art-20043897

Mayo Clinic Staff. (n.d.). Walking: Make it count with activity trackers. Mayo Clinic. https://www.mayoclinic.org/healthy-lifestyle/fitness/in-depth/walking/art-20047880

McCoy, J. (2019, January 3). *How to set realistic fitness goals you'll actually achieve, according to top trainers.* Self. https://www.self.com/story/how-to-set-realistic-fitness-goals

McGuire, R. (2014, October 22). *Woman athlete running exercise sprint cinder-track*. Pixabay. https://pixabay.com/photos/woman-athlete-running-exercise-498257/

McNeice, J. (2018, November 28). *The benefits of walking in nature*. Mind Matters Mental Health Training. https://www.mindmatterstraining.co.uk/benefits-walking-nature/

Most, J., & Redman, L. M. (2020). Impact of calorie restriction on energy metabolism in humans. *Experimental Gerontology, 133,* 110875. https://doi.org/10.1016/j.exger.2020.110875

Mueller, J. (2015, February 2). *8 strength training moves for walkers*. Spark People. https://www.sparkpeople.com/resource/fitness_articles.asp?id=2021

Neporent, L. (n.d.). *Structuring your walking program*. Dummies. https://www.dummies.com/health/exercise/structuring-your-walking-program/

Palinski-Wade, E. (n.d.). *Walking indoors*. Dummies. https://www.dummies.com/health/exercise/cardio/walking-indoors/

Pasja 1000. (2018, February 11). *Father lake river at the court of the seagulls*. Pixabay. https://pixabay.com/photos/father-lake-river-at-the-court-of-3144925/

Pexels. (2016, November 18). *House architecture front yard garage home*. Pixabay. https://pixabay.com/photos/house-architecture-front-yard-1836070/

REFERENCES

Physical inactivity a leading cause of disease and disability, warns WHO. (2002, April 4). World Health Organization. https://www.who.int/news/item/04-04-2002-physical-inactivity-a-leading-cause-of-disease-and-disability-warns-who

Rabbitt, M. (2020, July 15). *10 biggest benefits of walking to improve your health, according to experts.* Prevention. https://www.prevention.com/fitness/a20485587/benefits-from-walking-every-day/

Ring, F. (n.d.). *Weight loss benefits of interval walking – Increase your metabolism.* Walking For Health And Fitness. https://www.walkingforhealthandfitness.com/blog/weight-loss-benefits-of-interval-walking

Roland, J. (2020, January 16). *How to walk properly with good posture.* Healthline. https://www.healthline.com/health/how-to-walk

Russell-Jones, D., & Khan, R. (2007). Insulin-associated weight gain in diabetes – causes, effects and coping strategies. *Diabetes, Obesity and Metabolism, 9*(6), 799–812. https://doi.org/10.1111/j.1463-1326.2006.00686.x

Schroederhund. (2016, November 4). *Autumn walk autumn fall foliage fall color.* Pixabay. https://pixabay.com/photos/autumn-walk-autumn-fall-foliage-1792812/

Six-week beginner walking plan. (n.d.). American Heart Association.

https://www.heart.org/idc/groups/heart-public/@wcm/@fc/documents/downloadable/ucm_449261.pdf

Skjong, I., & Roberts, A. (2021, March 17). *The best fitness trackers.* The New York Times. https://www.nytimes.com/wirecutter/reviews/the-best-fitness-trackers/

Skwarecki, B. (2019, February 15). *How to track your food without counting calories.* Lifehacker. https://vitals.lifehacker.com/how-to-track-your-food-without-counting-calories-1832649187

Stables, J. (2021, March 30). *Best fitness tracker 2021: Top picks for all budgets.* Wareable. https://www.wareable.com/fitness-trackers/the-best-fitness-tracker

Steinhilber, B. (2018, May 4). *Why walking is the most underrated form of exercise.* NBC News. https://www.nbcnews.com/better/health/why-walking-most-underrated-form-exercise-ncna797271

StockSnap. (2017, August 6). *People man alone walking road tunnel travel sign.* Pixabay. https://pixabay.com/photos/people-man-alone-walking-road-2598817/

Tavrionov, M. (2017, October 21). *Glass water napkin sky reflection glass tumbler.* Pixabay. https://pixabay.com/photos/glass-water-napkin-sky-reflection-2875091/

Team Verywell. (2021, February 6). *Calculating the correct portion sizes for weight loss.* Verywell Fit. https://www.very-

REFERENCES

wellfit.com/proper-food-portion-sizes-for-weight-loss-3495475

Waehner, P. (2019, November 25). *Weight loss and fitness progress chart.* Verywell Fit. https://www.verywellfit.com/weight-loss-and-fitness-track-progress-chart-1231119

Waehner, P. (2020, January 21). *How to track your weight loss progress.* Verywell Fit. https://www.verywellfit.com/ways-to-track-weight-loss-progress-1231581

Walk your way to wellness. (n.d.). Chi Running. https://www.chirunning.com/chiwalking/walking-technique/

Walljasper, J. (2015, October 17). *Take a walk: 11 ways to build the healthy habit.* Yes Magazine. https://www.yesmagazine.org/health-happiness/2015/10/17/eleven-ways-built-healthy-habit-walking-vivek-murthy/

Weiner, Z. (2020, March 18). *Why it's important to do stretches before walking, no matter how many steps you're clocking.* Well And Good. https://www.wellandgood.com/stretches-before-walking/

What is rucking? (n.d.). Goruck. https://www.goruck.com/pages/what-is-rucking%20/

Why warming up and cooling down is important. (2016, December 15). Tri-City Medical Center. https://www.tricitymed.org/2016/12/warming-cooling-important/

REFERENCES

Wiggins, E. (2015, May 26). *Hiking for beginners: 10 essential tips*. Liftopia. https://blog.liftopia.com/10-essential-hiking-tips-beginner-hike/

Wikipedia Contributors. (2019, December 9). *Computer vision syndrome*. Wikipedia Foundation. https://en.wikipedia.org/wiki/Computer_vision_syndrome

Wikipedia Contributors. (2019, March 6). *Sedentary lifestyle*. Wikipedia Foundation. https://en.wikipedia.org/wiki/Sedentary_lifestyle

Wokandapix. (2017, June 6). *Plan objective strategy goal process success*. Pixabay. https://pixabay.com/photos/plan-objective-strategy-goal-2372176/

Www_slon_pics. (2017, May 2). *Despaired businessman business despair*. Pixabay. https://pixabay.com/photos/despaired-businessman-business-2261021/

INTERMITTENT FASTING FOR WOMEN

A GUIDE TO CREATING A SUSTAINABLE, LONG-TERM LIFESTYLE FOR WEIGHT LOSS AND BETTER HEALTH! INCLUDES HOW TO START, 16:8, 5:2, OMAD, FAST 800, ADM, WARRIOR AND FAST 5!

HEALTHFIT PUBLISHING

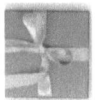 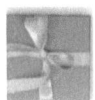

A Free Bonus To Our Readers

To get you started on your intermittent fasting journey, we have created

- 40 Low-Carb Recipes
- 35 Mediterranean Recipes
- 35 Keto Recipes
- A 31-Day Meal Plan

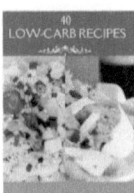 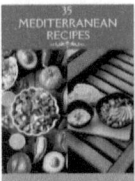 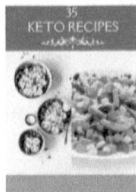 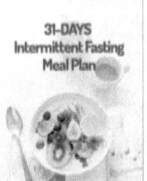

Free Bonus #1   Free Bonus #2   Free Bonus #3   Free Bonus #4

These 110 intermittent fasting recipes are delicious, healthy and easy to prepare. Each recipe includes serving sizes, nutritional data, and detailed step-by-step instructions. A weekly grocery shopping list is also included with the 31-Day Meal Plan.

To get your free bonuses, please click on the link or scan the QR code below and let us know the email address to send it to.

https://healthfitpublishing.com/bonus/iffw/

INTRODUCTION

"Healthy isn't a goal. It's a way of life."

— UNKNOWN

Weight loss isn't easy, but it is always possible. No matter who you are and your circumstances, you can lose weight if you want to. All you have to do is believe. Believing in yourself and your ability to lose weight is one of the greatest motivators. With proper motivation, successful weight loss is achievable; you are more likely to put in maximum effort and are less likely to throw in the towel.

Women are especially placed under pressure to conform to societal expectations. These expectations are often unrealistic and unfair but they're there nonetheless. On top of societal pressure, there is more and more research emerging to connect carrying extra weight with health conditions such as diabetes and heart disease. To make matters worse, the moment women hit perimenopause, their bodies turn traitor and the number on the scale seems to inevitably creep up.

Transforming your life may seem like an insurmountable task. There are countless people who have done it before and succeeded, and they didn't do it with crash diets. What they did do is lose weight at a healthy rate and they learned how to keep it off. Superfast yo-yo crash dieting may be alluring for its speedy results. However, it has been proven that this type of success doesn't last. What you want is a sustainable lifestyle change that will help you to shed the pounds and inches and keep them off. Guess what? It's easier than you think.

Optimal health starts with what you fuel your body with – your diet – but that's not all. It's not just about what you eat. Your eating patterns – when you eat – can have a significant impact on weight loss and how your body uses the fuel available to it.

"A healthy outside starts from the inside."

Robert Urich

INTRODUCTION

Changing when you fuel your body is the first step toward creating a healthy body and happy life. However, simply changing when you eat isn't enough to ensure you are healthy and shed those pesky pounds. You need to enjoy a delicious, healthy diet as well to ensure your body is properly nourished. An inadequately nourished body isn't going to adapt to an intermittent fasting lifestyle well and could lead you to give up when you really shouldn't.

The consumption of fast food, artificial ingredients, added salt and sugar, and many other aspects of a typical modern Western diet are detrimental to your health. Their flavors were created to tempt you into buying them, lining the pockets of big processed food corporations, irrespective of the health complications these foods can cause. One major health concern is the constantly rising rate of obesity worldwide.

A healthy diet can be just as tasty as junk food, if not more so, and offers you the nutrition you need to improve your health, increase your energy, curb excessive calorie intake, and even burn fat for weight loss.

Your eating patterns can also influence your health and weight loss. At first glance, intermittent fasting may seem daunting and even impossible. It may go against the grain of what you currently think you know about diet and lifestyle. After all, how can going for hours on end without eating be good for you? This is where believing outdated concepts is keeping you from enjoying a healthy lifestyle and achieving

INTRODUCTION

sustainable weight loss. Fasting is easier than you think. We're going to tell you why and how to do it easily and safely.

Within the pages of this book lies a wealth of knowledge compiled to help you live your best, healthiest, and happiest life. We are going to:

- Introduce you to intermittent fasting, telling you why and how it works.
- Provide you with several popular fasting methods.
- Give advice on how to get started, including some tips and tricks to make it easier.
- Tell you why a healthy diet is so important, which diet is the healthiest and easiest to follow in the world, and how to adopt it.

As a bonus to help you achieve a holistically healthy lifestyle, we'll also:

- Explain walking as the best, most effective form of exercise for a wide range of people, irrespective of age and some physical limitations.
- Provide you with compelling reasons to get fit and explain how to incorporate other forms of exercise into your walks to maximize the benefits.

In a nutshell, we are going to help you transform your life, achieve your weight loss goals, and adopt a healthy, happy lifestyle through simple changes. Once you experience the life-changing benefits of combining intermittent fasting, a healthy diet, and exercise, you're never going to look back.

Are you ready to reclaim your health, life, and happiness?

ABOUT HEALTHFIT PUBLISHING

Healthfit Publishing is a health and wellness publishing brand. Our mission is to bring sound, actionable knowledge and advice straight from the health and wellness industry to readers from all walks of life. Our focus is on simple lifestyle changes that are easy to make for improving your overall quality of life.

We are made up of a diverse group of dynamic individuals who are passionate about inspiring and motivating others to achieve their health, fitness, and weight loss goals. Our team members are well-respected in their fields and bring expertise and experience in wellness, health, fitness, nutrition, and meticulous research to the table. We are dedicated to making healthy living accessible to anyone who is interested in transforming their life and boosting their happiness by improving their wellbeing.

Our team's diversity is our strong point and the common thread that brings us together is a zest for living life to its fullest and a passion for healthy living. Exercise and good nutrition are just two of our top interests and it's not hard to find inspiration in either.

PART I

ALL ABOUT INTERMITTENT FASTING

1

THE WHAT, WHY, AND HOW OF INTERMITTENT FASTING

Intermittent fasting has made a bold appearance on the diet and health scene in recent times. While it has grown exponentially in popularity in the past few years, it's not a here-today-gone-tomorrow health craze that the next fad diet will easily replace. Intermittent fasting is a real, viable healthy lifestyle change that has been proven to work. Look at how many people engage in intermittent fasting, and not just for short periods. Intermittent fasting works so well for many people that they successfully stick to the fasting lifestyle for months and even years.

Let's delve deeper into fasting, and specifically the practice of intermittent fasting, to show you why it works, how it works, and what it can do for you.

WHAT IS FASTING?

Fasting is the practice of forgoing food or drink, and sometimes both, for a period of time. There are many reasons people fast, ranging from cultural and spiritual practices, to health reasons. Fasting doesn't necessarily come down to a hard-and-fast rule of abstaining from food or drink completely. While there is full fasting, where you can either eat and/or drink nothing at all, there is also partial fasting, where certain limitations are placed on how much you can eat. Fasting periods also vary depending on the reason for fasting and can range from several hours to even a few days.

Intermittent fasting may seem to be a relatively new kid on the block, but the concept of using fasting for therapeutic or medicinal reasons has been around since as far back as the fifth century BC. Hippocrates, an ancient Greek physician, was the first to advocate fasting as a medicinal treatment for a variety of ailments.

The medical world turned its attention back to fasting for therapeutic and medicinal benefits of weight loss in the 1960s and since then, more and more research has been done on the practice. With the advancement of medical technology, our understanding of the human body and its nutritional requirements has vastly improved and expanded since the turn of the twentieth century. Due to this renewed interest and increasing research into the benefits of fasting, our approach to fasting has been honed to develop an effective lifestyle for health and weight loss.

WHAT IS INTERMITTENT FASTING?

Intermittent fasting is mistakenly seen as a diet, but it's far from the typical concept of one. The focus of intermittent fasting isn't on what you eat. While a healthy, balanced diet is encouraged to maximize the benefits of the practice, intermittent fasting is concerned with when you eat. It is essentially an eating pattern that schedules an eating period, also known as an "eating window", between periods of fasting.

An example of an intermittent fasting plan is the 18:6 method. When practicing this method, you cycle between eighteen hours of fasting and a six-hour eating window. Once your eating window has ended, it's back to fasting for another 18 hours. The periods of fasting are variable, depending on the method you choose to follow. This is just one example of an intermittent fasting plan and we'll tell you all about the other most popular methods and how to do them in a later chapter.

To reap the rewards of adopting an intermittent fasting lifestyle, proper nutrition and calorie control are essential. The effects will be greatly diminished, if not negated altogether, by making poor food choices and eating too much during your eating window. Consuming too many calories, irrespective of when you consume them, still represents a higher energy intake than energy expenditure, which won't lead to weight loss.

Intermittent fasting can take on various forms, as there is no one way to do it. Your fasting can range from several hours to an entire day. Because of this variety, the fasting lifestyle appeals to a wide spectrum of people, since you may choose and tailor a plan that works for you. We'll explain just how to do it and how to choose the right schedule to meet your needs in a later section of this book. For now, let's look at how and why intermittent fasting works.

INTERMITTENT FASTING: HOW IT WORKS

Intermittent fasting is effective because your body enters a fasted state, which may also put your body into the metabolic state of ketosis. You're not only impacting your calorie burn when you're fasting; you're also influencing your hormones. Hormonal changes are the key to intermittent fasting's success, so let's take a closer look at what being in a fasted state means and how it affects your hormones.

Your Body in a Fasted State

Intermittent fasting goes against the grain of typical modern human eating schedules or patterns. Today, a typical human eating pattern involves eating regularly throughout your waking hours. In times gone by, a healthy, balanced diet and regular eating schedule can be beneficial for weight management and maintaining a healthy weight. However, in our modern world, a sedentary lifestyle has largely become the norm, which adversely affects health.

Office jobs and technological advancements in entertainment see you sitting down most of your waking hours. You then go to sleep at night. The total daily activity of the "average Joe" on the street has decreased dramatically and you need physical activity to burn off the calories you eat. Another problem is that too many of us are consuming an increasingly unhealthy diet that is high in non-nutritive calories. Your body is likely to be getting more calories than it needs and, at the same time, not getting proper nutrition to keep it functioning optimally.

Weight loss requires consuming fewer calories than your body burns in a day. When calorie intake exceeds daily calorie burn, you have weight gain. Weight maintenance occurs when your calorie intake and energy expenditure match up.

When you eat, most food is broken down into sugars which are then used as fuel for your body. Excess sugar is stored in your muscles to be used when blood sugar drops. Further excess sugar is stored as fat reserves for when your blood sugar and muscle sugar stores are depleted. When you don't eat for several hours, your body enters a fasted state in which blood sugar is used up and muscle sugar stores are depleted. When this takes place, your body is forced to burn fat to keep going.

Intermittent fasting is effective because it prolongs the hours in which your body has no choice but to burn fat for fuel. When you follow a regular eating schedule, your body won't burn fat continuously or as effectively, even on a low-calorie diet, because of a regular influx of sugar.

It takes approximately eight to twelve hours after your last meal for your body to deplete its sugar stores, enter a fasted state, and start burning fat.

Hormones: The Intermittent Fasting Effect

As you now know, intermittent fasting influences your hormones. There are several key hormones that are affected when your body goes into a fasted state. Taking a more in-depth look at each key hormone, how they typically work, and how fasting affects them will offer a greater understanding of exactly why and how this lifestyle works.

Insulin

Insulin is the first and foremost affected hormone when you are fasting. Here's the role it plays in your body and how intermittent fasting affects it:

- Food is eaten and broken down into sugars which are released into your bloodstream, signaling insulin release.
- Insulin transports the sugar throughout your body to be used.

- Once you are fully fueled, excess sugar is converted into glycogen and stored in your muscles for later use when blood sugar runs low.
- Once glycogen stores are full, further excess sugar is converted to fat and stored.
- Fasting prolongs the period of time for which your body doesn't need insulin, which helps to prevent insulin resistance and promote weight loss.

Glucagon

Glucagon does the opposite job of insulin:

- When blood sugar levels decrease, glucagon is released.
- Stored glycogen is retrieved and converted into sugar for energy.
- Fasting lowers your blood sugar, stimulating glucagon release, leading to depleted glycogen stores.
- Fat is burned for energy when glycogen stores are depleted, aiding weight loss.

Ghrelin

Ghrelin is your hunger hormone. It is released to stimulate hunger as a cue to eat. Ghrelin is typically released in accordance with your regular eating patterns. Fasting changes your eating schedule and your body has to adapt, rescheduling ghrelin release accordingly. This adjustment period is what causes hunger pangs during the early stages of entering a fasting lifestyle. These hunger pangs will lessen as your body adjusts.

Leptin

Leptin is produced by fat cells. This hormone regulates appetite. The amount of leptin generated is proportional to the amount of body fat you have. Increased leptin levels should suppress your appetite.

Leptin resistance may develop from excessive leptin production. Excessive leptin levels desensitize your body and brain to the appetite-suppressing effects of leptin. This results in feeling less satisfied after a meal, leading to overeating and weight gain.

Fasting aids in the loss of body fat, decreasing leptin production, and lowering your risk of developing leptin resistance. Decreased leptin levels may even re-sensitize your body to its effects.

Adiponectin

Fasting aids the loss of body fat, which decreases leptin production and increases appetite, but it also increases levels of adiponectin. Adiponectin is a hormonal powerhouse that:

- regulates how fats and sugars are used
- aids in burning body fat
- reduces inflammation in your body

- reduces the build-up of cholesterol in your arteries

Human Growth Hormone (HGH)

The human growth hormone plays a role both in building lean muscle mass and in the breakdown of fat. There are three things that stimulate your body to increase the release of human growth hormone:

- getting enough sleep
- exercise
- low blood sugar levels

Higher insulin levels suppress the release of the human growth hormone. Fasting lowers blood sugar, decreases insulin levels, and increases human growth hormone release.

The benefit of HGH's promotion of lean muscle mass is that increased lean muscle burns more calories naturally. The combination of fat-burning and muscle-growth effects of the human growth hormone makes it a powerful ally in transforming your body on your weight loss journey.

IS INTERMITTENT FASTING HEALTHY AND SAFE?

Most people can safely practice intermittent fasting. Not only that, but research is supporting a variety of health benefits that you can enjoy while following an intermittent fasting program. For over 1,000 years, people have practiced fasting for a variety of purposes. Fasting is still widely practiced for cultural and religious reasons today, with no negative consequences for the millions of people who undertake it around the world.

However, there are certain people who shouldn't fast and you should always get the all-clear from your doctor before starting a program like intermittent fasting.

WHO SHOULDN'T PRACTICE INTERMITTENT FASTING?

Intermittent fasting is associated with a long list of health benefits and it's generally safe to do. Weight loss is one of the most popular reasons for taking up intermittent fasting. This is all well and good, but there are situations in which you shouldn't practice fasting for any period of time. Intermittent fasting could be unsafe or unsuitable if you fall into one of the following categories:

Diabetics

Having diabetes means that you constantly have a high level of sugar in your blood. Intermittent fasting has been shown to affect blood sugar levels. During your fasting period, your blood glucose levels drop, which might sound like an ideal solution if you have diabetes. However, intermittent fasting isn't a solution to high blood sugar levels, unless it's done in a controlled and supervised way. You should not fast if your blood sugar levels are unstable, you have difficulty regulating your blood sugar, you have been diagnosed as diabetic, or you use any type of medication to help you balance your blood sugar.

If you are already taking diabetes medicine that reduces your blood sugar, reducing it further during fasting times may be risky. Your blood sugar could be at risk of dropping to an unhealthily low level. The same could happen if you experience unstable blood sugar. Blood sugar levels that are too low put you at risk of shakiness, dizziness, fainting, or even entering a coma.

The second danger of fasting as a diabetic is that it may cause blood sugar level spikes. After periods of fasting, eating could cause your blood sugar to rise to dangerous levels. The risk is increased when breaking your fast with carbohydrate-rich food or if fasting leads to overeating.

People Taking Medication

Both intermittent fasting and some types of medication influence your body's hormones. The two could interact badly with each other if you take up intermittent fasting while you are taking medication. Not all medication will interact negatively with fasting, but it's better to be safe than sorry. Before beginning an intermittent fasting program, check with your doctor to see if fasting will interact with your medication.

Underweight Individuals

One of the primary reasons to begin intermittent fasting is for the weight loss benefits connected with your body using fat for fuel while fasting. However, if you are underweight or trying to gain weight, intermittent fasting isn't for you. It may be a generally healthy eating pattern, but it's going to have the opposite effect to the healthy weight gain that you are aiming for.

If you are underweight, you don't have much body fat, so losing some of it could send your body into distress. Having too little body fat could cause complications such as amenorrhea (loss of monthly menstruation) and fertility problems. Women experience amenorrhea in two drastically different instances of having very little body fat. Both anorexia sufferers and top athletes may experience the loss of their monthly cycle. The difference is that athletes are incredibly healthy and not underweight.

There is an additional risk posed to someone who has very little body fat. When your body fat drops very low, you are at risk of a process called catabolism, also known as "muscle wasting", where your body starts to 'eat' its own muscle. Your body does this in response to having very little fat to burn. It breaks down your muscle tissue, essentially cannibalizing itself, for fuel. You will start to lose muscle mass across the board and that includes the potential of damaging your heart. Your heart is called "the love muscle" for a reason; it's made of muscle and is just as susceptible to catabolism as any other muscle in your body.

Important note: If you are naturally slim, but not sure whether you are underweight or not and want to practice intermittent fasting for health reasons apart from weight loss, consult a doctor. A doctor will be able to examine your physical health to determine whether you are underweight or if fasting is safe, considering that you are likely to lose some weight.

Those with Current or Past Disordered Eating Habits

If you currently suffer from an eating disorder or are recovering from one, intermittent fasting is not a safe practice for you. Even if you suffered from an eating disorder in the past and have since fully recovered, it still may not be safe to fast. Fasting may put you at risk of continuing or redeveloping unhealthy eating patterns.

Intermittent fasting is more than just a physical experience. It is also a mental experience. Having such current or past unhealthy mental food relationships puts you at risk of relapsing and falling back into old habits.

Anyone who has been bulimic in the past may be at risk of relapsing into binge-eating after their fasting period is over each day. Anyone who has suffered anorexia in the past may be tempted to take fasting to the limit and beyond, falling back into unhealthily restrictive eating habits and consuming too little food, too infrequently.

Those Trying to Conceive or with Fertility Issues

As we know, intermittent fasting affects your body's hormones. Many of the effects are positive, but the fertility hormones that regulate your menstrual cycle could be negatively influenced. Intermittent fasting might suppress certain hormones, which could cause irregular ovulation or even the possibility of a complete cessation of ovulation. Intermittent fasting isn't for you if you are trying to have a baby.

The reason intermittent fasting could suppress ovulation is that your body may not feel that the circumstances are right for bearing a child and therefore it will suppress the hormones necessary to stimulate ovulation. No ovulation means no menstruation. The whole reason women have a menstrual cycle is to prepare the womb for ovulation, to ovulate, and then to menstruate to remove the prepared womb lining and unfertilized ovum. There is no need to prepare the womb or menstruate if there is no ovulation.

Pregnant Women

Pregnancy and fasting simply don't go together. Intermittent fasting is popular for weight loss, but there is no good reason to try to lose weight while pregnant, even if you were overweight before falling pregnant. Every expecting mother should expect to put on a little bit of baby weight while pregnant.

Intermittent fasting has been demonstrated to reduce blood sugar and blood pressure. Lowering both blood pressure and blood sugar regularly during pregnancy could be detrimental to the healthy growth and development of your baby.

Breastfeeding Women

While your baby is breastfeeding, they are entirely dependent on your breast milk to meet their nutritional needs during a crucial time in their growth and development. Even if you pair intermittent fasting with a healthy, balanced diet, you may experience disruptions to your milk supply which would leave your baby in the lurch.

The other consideration to take into account is that your caloric needs are higher than normal while breastfeeding. You may unwittingly consume too few calories for your body's needs due to the inclination to naturally consume fewer calories during a shortened eating window.

Women with a History of Amenorrhea

As you are now keenly aware, intermittent fasting has an effect on female hormones, specifically those related to fertility and menstruation. Amenorrhea refers to a woman having an irregular menstrual cycle and missing her period occasionally or for long stretches of time. Intermittent fasting could induce amenorrhea more easily in individuals who have a history of amenorrhea or it could worsen the problem.

Those with Sugar Retention Problems

Sugar retention refers to your body's ability to hold onto and use the sugars from your food to provide your body with energy. Intermittent fasting lowers your blood sugar levels. When you have issues with retaining sugar, lowered blood sugar levels could pose a problem. Due to a shortened eating window and the natural tendency to consume fewer calories during that shortened window, you could also fail to take in enough carbohydrates to fuel your body.

Individuals with Low Blood Pressure

Intermittent fasting affects various functions and aspects of your body. One of these aspects is blood pressure. Fasting has the effect of reducing blood pressure, which can be beneficial if your blood pressure is high. If you already have low blood pressure, however, decreasing it even more by adopting intermittent fasting could cause serious complications.

ALWAYS CHECK WITH YOUR DOCTOR

Before you embark upon a weight loss journey to transform your body and improve your life through intermittent fasting, it is imperative that you consult your family doctor. Only a qualified medical professional can perform a full physical examination to determine whether the big changes will be safe for you. Intermittent fasting is a serious lifestyle change. You are drastically altering your eating patterns and retraining your body to thrive on alternating periods of fasting and eating. Even if you think it is a safe change to make, it's better to be safe than sorry. It's wise to let your doctor know about your plans. It is possible that your doctor could even offer you advice on what method of intermittent fasting would be most suitable.

THE BOTTOM LINE

Intermittent fasting is not a new concept. It is a generally safe practice, but you should always consult your family doctor before starting a fasting program. Fasting is a practical way to lose weight and now you know just how it can help you to achieve your goal of shedding unwanted pounds. Plus, you now know what happens to your body in a fasted state and who shouldn't fast.

Next up, we'll discuss the myriad of health benefits associated with intermittent fasting.

2

WHY CHOOSE INTERMITTENT FASTING?

Intermittent fasting offers a wealth of health benefits. These benefits are what make it a popular lifestyle choice for those wanting to improve their health. What will intermittent fasting do for you that is so wonderful? Let's examine the benefits it provides and how it does so.

WEIGHT LOSS

One of the most popular reasons that people take up intermittent fasting as a healthy lifestyle choice is for weight loss. How does intermittent fasting achieve this?

- As your body becomes accustomed to your new eating patterns and shortened eating windows, there is a tendency to naturally consume fewer calories during the shorter space of time in which you can eat. Eating fewer calories helps to create a calorie deficit and we all know that to lose weight, calories coming in should be less than calories going out. When your body doesn't have enough calories to fuel its functions and maintain your weight at the same time, it will start to access your fat reserves for energy.

- Fasting for periods of time lowers your blood sugar levels, stimulating the production of hormones needed to convert fat into ketones for energy.
- Lowering your blood sugar levels automatically lowers your insulin levels and stimulates the production of human growth hormone which aids in converting fat into energy.
- Lower insulin levels prevent your body from converting and storing sugars as fat.
- When practicing intermittent fasting, you are likely to lose less lean muscle mass than on a typical weight loss diet. Maintaining your lean muscle and helping increase it through the production of HGH helps to keep your metabolism from slowing as much as it may otherwise while following a regular weight loss diet.

INTERMITTENT FASTING MAY BE EASIER THAN TRADITIONAL DIETING

Typical dieting – in the sense of adopting a diet that is low in carbohydrates, fat, sodium, and sugar – or any conventional diet associated with weight loss, may seem easier than fasting. The thought of fasting for hours at a time may seem like it would be really hard, but the truth is that you may find it an easier option.

When you adopt a typical weight loss diet, it generally involves restricting the foods you enjoy. You may feel deprived of foods, which could cause and amplify cravings for them. It also fosters a deprivation mindset, making dieting seem like personal torture and increasing your chances of giving in to cravings and cheating or quitting your diet entirely.

When you think about intermittent fasting, it may seem impossible. The thought of a prolonged period of time without food seems difficult. In reality, fasting may actually be easier than you think. The idea of fighting cravings may seem less daunting, especially when you believe you have the willpower to resist those cravings.

The thought of hunger may seem more challenging, but, in actual fact, your body adjusts to your new eating schedule and it becomes easier over time. Once your body adjusts, you aren't hungry all the time and you don't feel deprived of your favorite foods, because you can still enjoy them in moderation during your eating windows.

"Diets are easy in the contemplation, difficult in the execution. Intermittent fasting is just the opposite – it's difficult in the contemplation, but easy in the execution. – Dr. Michael Eades

METABOLISM

Do you remember reading that intermittent fasting has an effect on your human growth hormone which helps maintain lean muscle mass? Loss of fat and muscle is an inevitable part of any weight loss journey, but how you go about losing weight can influence how much lean body mass you lose.

There are two aspects of intermittent fasting that offer you an advantage over regular dieting. First, intermittent fasting maintains more of your lean muscle during weight loss than other, traditional types of weight loss diets. Second, severe calorie restrictions are also not necessary for weight loss by practicing fasting. The combination of preserving more lean muscle and milder calorie restrictions helps to improve your metabolism.

During a typical diet, calories are often greatly restricted, and over time, your body cottons on to what is happening and slows your metabolism down accordingly, to make the most of the energy from your food. Intermittent fasting, on the other hand, helps to burn fat by depleting your sugar stores and then using fat for energy, before you refuel when you break your fast.

Across several days, you are not restricting your calorie intake as much as with typical dieting, but rather, you're encouraging your body to burn fat in between eating windows. You are essentially bypassing your body's natural tendency to slow your metabolism down in the face of excessive calorie restriction.

This combination of tricking your body into maintaining your metabolism and preserving more muscle (which also contributes to maintaining the rate of metabolism) makes fasting a better option for effective, healthy weight loss.

TYPE 2 DIABETES AND INSULIN RESISTANCE

As we learned in the previous chapter, insulin resistance develops due to a constant influx of sugar from carbohydrate-rich food. Your blood sugar levels are kept high and your body is continually trying to combat the high blood sugar by stimulating your pancreas to produce insulin. After some time of constantly being bombarded with insulin, the cells in your body become desensitized to it and your pancreas just can't keep up with the demand. Your blood sugar levels will remain consistently high and may even begin to rise as a result of the insulin's decreasing effectiveness over time. This is the time to do something about the problem – before it gets out of control and develops into prediabetes.

Prediabetes is a condition caused by higher than normal blood sugar levels that are not yet high enough to be classified as diabetes. If left untreated, prediabetes develops into type 2 diabetes when the blood sugar levels reach an unhealthy level. If type 2 diabetes is left unchecked, it will eventually develop into the more serious type 1 diabetes, which may require medical intervention to control. Nobody wants that to happen.

Intermittent fasting helps to prevent or even reverse insulin resistance, the first link in the diabetes chain. When your body enters a fasted state, your blood sugar levels decrease and so too does your insulin level.

Reduced insulin levels in the body could help to increase your sensitivity to insulin, making it more effective at removing sugar from your bloodstream when you do break your fast.

CELLULAR REPAIR

The rate at which your body repairs damaged cells and replaces them with new, healthy cells is increased by intermittent fasting. During fasting, there is less energy from sugar to go around and your cells start to feel the pressure. To make the most of the energy that is available through burning fat, your body starts to weed out damaged cells. After all, if they are damaged and not working properly, they represent an unnecessary drain on the energy supply.

Your body starts to metabolize those unhealthy cells and replaces them with new, healthy cells. Unhealthy cells using energy to do a half-job are energy inefficient, whereas healthy cells using vital energy to perform properly are more energy efficient. Thus, your rate of cellular repair is increased when your body is in a fasted state.

SLOWING AGING

Nobody likes to feel the effects of aging and intermittent fasting helps to slow this process down. Aging is basically the result of damage to your body over time. It starts degenerating, which is why people develop all sorts of problems as they get older, such as reduced mobility.

Part of the aging process is exposure to oxidative stress caused by free radicals. Free radicals are particles within your body that cause damage to your body's cells. Intermittent fasting helps to reduce the number of free radicals floating around your body and therefore reduces the amount of damage they can do. Less damage from free radicals means a slower rate of aging.

INFLAMMATION AND DISEASE

Intermittent fasting increases the rate of cellular repair, which helps to combat aging, but that's not all it helps with. A higher rate of cellular repair also helps to ease inflammation and combat the effects of certain diseases, including degenerative diseases and cancer.

Inflammation occurs when cells – or groups of cells called tissues – in your body are damaged in some way. Having lots of free radicals floating around doing further damage doesn't help. However, intermittent fasting comes to the rescue again. By reducing the number of free radicals and encouraging your body to repair damaged cells more quickly, fasting helps to reduce inflammation and speeds up healing.

Degenerative disease is mitigated by reducing the damage done by free radicals and by increasing cellular repair. The faster damaged cells are repaired or replaced, the better you will feel. The advancement of degenerative disease is effectively slowed down.

Important note: Intermittent fasting isn't a cure-all for disease and it isn't guaranteed to completely reverse the effects of degenerative disease. What it will do is help slow the progression down, improving your quality of life.

Let's take a look at cancer, another form of degenerative disease, and how intermittent fasting influences your risk of developing cancer.

The first way in which fasting helps to lower your risk of cancer is through weight loss. Obesity has been associated to a number of cancers, including:

- Breast cancer
- Colorectal cancer
- Esophageal cancer
- Gallbladder cancer
- Head and neck cancer
- Pancreatic cancer
- Prostate cancer
- Thyroid cancer
- Uterine cancer

Obesity-related cancers are less likely to develop if you maintain a healthy weight. What about other cancers though? To understand how intermittent fasting helps to reduce your risk of developing cancer, you need to understand what cancer is.

Cancer develops when cells in your body become damaged and dysfunctional. These abnormal cells proceed to divide and multiply out of control, causing a tumor, and can spread to other parts of your body where they do the same thing. The increased rate of cellular repair encouraged by intermittent fasting means that unhealthy cells are removed faster, giving them less time to develop into something more serious. This increased removal of damaged and dysfunctional cells lowers your risk of unhealthy cells getting out of control and developing into cancerous growths.

Important note: Intermittent fasting does not cure or specifically prevent the development of cancer. It is simply a recommended lifestyle, as it may lower your risk. Remember that other factors may raise your risk, such as smoking, alcohol abuse, unhealthy diet, and even genetics.

HEART HEALTH

Intermittent fasting influences the way your body metabolizes sugar and cholesterol. It decreases low-density lipoprotein, or bad cholesterol, to lower your total cholesterol level by raising the proportion of good cholesterol to bad cholesterol in your bloodstream. Improving your cholesterol helps to reduce your risk of developing cardiovascular disease, making intermittent fasting a heart-healthy lifestyle choice.

Intermittent fasting reduces your risk of heart disease by encouraging weight loss and healthy weight maintenance. Maintaining a healthy weight lowers your insulin levels and reduces your risk of developing diabetes. Both obesity and diabetes are linked to cardiovascular disease. Lowering your risks adds up to a reduced risk of heart health problems.

BRAIN HEALTH

Brain health is influenced by several factors, all of which are improved by intermittent fasting:

- Blood pressure
- Blood sugar levels
- Inflammation
- Insulin resistance
- Oxidative stress from free radicals

Improving these aspects of your health will automatically improve brain function, but that's not all. Intermittent fasting is linked to:

- The formation of new neural nerve cells
- Improved memory
- Increased levels of healthy brain hormones
- Ketosis in a fasted state, which increases the number of energy-producing mitochondria in the brain, offering better fuel for your brain than sugar

THE BOTTOM LINE

So, now you know why you should choose intermittent fasting. It offers a whole host of health benefits that you simply cannot turn down.

The next step is choosing your intermittent fasting program. In the next chapter, we will discuss several fasting plans you can choose from, according to your personal needs.

3

POPULAR TYPES OF INTERMITTENT FASTING

Unlike other, more traditional diets such as low-carb diets, there isn't just one way to practice intermittent fasting. Due to the growing popularity of intermittent fasting, it has evolved to encompass a variety of methods. As such, it doesn't come in a one-size-fits-all format and offers several options to choose from to suit individual needs and preferences.

Some plans are customizable, further adding to their appeal, and some plans have been proven to be easier to adopt and maintain, while others are more difficult to get used to. If your ultimate goal is a more difficult type of intermittent fasting, you can start with an easier method and work your way up to the plan you want to adopt in the long term.

Important note: Not all of the following fasting methods will be the most suitable options for women. Please read Chapter 4, which is specifically aimed at discussing the effects of fasting on women, before starting your fasting lifestyle.

Let's get started by discussing several different intermittent fasting methods so you can choose the option that is best for you.

16:8 METHOD: MOST POPULAR

Often called the 16:8 plan, 16:8 diet, or 16:8 method, and less commonly referred to as the lean gains method, this intermittent fasting method is considered to be the most popular and the easiest daily fasting plan to maintain in the long term. As the name suggests, on the 16:8 plan, you fast for sixteen hours of the day and have an eight-hour eating window.

How to Implement the 16:8 Method

One of the best things about this method is the flexibility to schedule your fasting periods and eating windows according to your personal schedule. Human beings are diurnal creatures, meaning that we are most active during daylight hours. Scheduling your eight-hour eating window is generally best done in the middle section of the day, so that it most closely resembles a typical daytime eating period. This allows your body to adjust more easily to a fasting plan, as it aligns with your natural internal clock, your circadian rhythm.

Having a gap of at least two to four hours after eating before going to sleep is suggested to have health benefits, as it allows your body to digest the food before it slows down at the end of the day. While sleeping, all your body functions slow to a snail's pace, allowing your body to achieve maximum rest. Going to sleep on a full stomach could result in acid reflux from your stomach, heartburn, and poor sleep quality. Following the 16:8 method, you can schedule your last meal well before bedtime to allow at least partial digestion.

It's Customizable

The customizable nature of the 16:8 plan is another part of its appeal. It offers daily flexibility to adjust eating window times to suit your needs on any given day. It isn't a rigid plan where the start and end times of your fasting period are set in stone, unlike some other fasting plans.

You can also customize your plan in accordance with your experience of fasting. If you have never fasted before, you can start with a shorter fasting period and build yourself up to longer periods. You can also fast for longer lengths of time once you've become accustomed to fasting. The variability of your fasting schedule is entirely up to you.

Possible variations of the 16:8 intermittent fasting method include:

- 12:12 – fasting for twelve hours with a twelve-hour eating window
- 14:10 – fasting for fourteen hours with a ten-hour eating window
- 16:8 – fasting for sixteen hours with an eight-hour eating window

Given that it takes your body around eight hours to attain a fasted state, you should try to fast for a minimum of 12 hours to start getting the benefits of fasting. It's also better to start off with a shorter fasting period and a longer eating window. That way, it's not a huge shock to your body.

THE FAST 5 METHOD

The Fast 5 Method is also known as the 19:5 method. It is similar to the 16:8 approach, except that the fasting phase is longer. Remember, the longer your fasting period, the longer you are keeping your body in mild ketosis and therefore the longer you're burning fat for fuel.

5:2 METHOD: EASIEST FOR STARTING FASTING

Also referred to as the fast diet, the 5:2 method is one of the easiest fasting plans to implement. If you feel intimidated by long, hard-and-fast periods without eating, this is the plan for you to use to get you on the road to the fasting lifestyle.

The 5:2 method may also be the best option for women who want to get into intermittent fasting.

How to Implement the 5:2 Method

Unlike the 16:8 method, the name of this fasting plan is a little more deceptive. It doesn't refer to an hour ratio, but rather to days. It is the springboard on which the Fast 800 plan was launched, and we'll get into the Fast 800 method next.

The 5:2 method isn't a solid fasting plan. Not all intermittent fasting plans involve not eating at all. Part of the ease of implementing this method is that you don't go completely without food for a whole day. Instead, you choose two fasting days per week and for the other five days, you eat a regular, healthy, and balanced diet.

When practicing this method, you restrict your calorie intake to 500 calories per fasting day. You can break your 500 calories up however you like, as small snacks throughout the day, two or three small meals, or even a single meal.

Another appealing aspect of the 5:2 plan is that it is entirely flexible. You don't have to fast for the same two days every week. You can decide on which days to fast and which to eat normally, according to your preference and social schedule. If you have a get-together, such as a meal with family or friends or even a work function, you can swap your fasting days around to accommodate those events. The only other requirement of this fasting plan is that there is at least one non-fasting day between your two fasting days.

FAST 800

The Fast 800 method is a stricter intermittent fasting plan than the 5:2 method and it consists of three stages. Again, as with the 5:2 method, the Fast 800 doesn't involve abstaining from food altogether.

Stage 1: Very Fast 800

This is stage one of the plan. It aims to achieve fast weight loss by restricting your daily caloric intake to 800 calories for a minimum of two weeks. However, should you feel that you are able to continue with this stage of the plan, you can maintain it for up to a maximum of 12 weeks. How long you maintain this stage of the plan is entirely up to you and depends on how comfortable you are and what your weight loss goals are.

It is important to eat a nutritious diet of foods that will help you feel satisfied longer. Foods that help you maintain satiety longer include whole foods and whole grains. Maintaining this kind of extremely low-calorie diet for an extended period of time can prove difficult in comparison to the typical 5:2 method mentioned above and, therefore, it isn't everyone's cup of tea.

Stage 2: The New 5:2

This is the second stage of the Fast 800 program. Based on the 5:2 plan, you are fasting for two days per week and eating normally for the other five days. However long you maintain the Very Fast 800 stage of the plan, this stage immediately follows that period. As with the original 5:2 approach, this second stage gives you the option of which two days of the week to fast, as long as there is at least one non-fasting day scheduled in between.

This stage of the plan has no time constraints. You can stay on this plan until you reach your weight loss goals. You can maintain this plan indefinitely. You could also use this stage of the plan as a stepping stone to other intermittent fasting methods. It is entirely up to you.

Stage 3: Way of Life

The second stage that we just looked at has no time limit and can be maintained indefinitely. However, if you decide that you no longer want to practice intermittent fasting or you are only using this fasting program for initial weight loss, you will reach the third stage, which is essentially a maintenance plan. All this means is following a healthy, balanced, and calorie-conscious diet going forward to maintain a healthy weight after shedding unwanted pounds.

ADM

The acronym ADM stands for the Alternate Day Method. The name is self-explanatory and it may also be called the 1:1 plan. This method is often considered to be one of the hardest intermittent fasting plans to follow in the long term and is difficult to start off with, even though you don't abstain from food completely. One probable explanation for this is that your body doesn't have a chance to adjust to a new eating schedule, since you're switching it up daily.

Using the Alternate Day Method, you will fast by restricting your calorie intake one day and eat normally every other day, cycling between fasting and non-fasting days. How much you restrict your calorie intake is up to you.

It is easier to embark upon this intermittent fasting plan by starting with a smaller restriction and gradually increasing the restriction on fasting days. You can use the original 5:2 method or the Fast 800 method as guidelines of how many calories you eat on fasting days. You can restrict to as little as between 500 and 800 calories.

EAT STOP EAT

The Eat Stop Eat method may sound exactly like the ADM, but there is a major difference between the two. Unlike the 1:1 ratio of the ADM, the Eat Stop Eat plan paces fasting days further out so that there are two non-fasting days between each fasting day. This gives you two to three fasting days per week. You will have two fasting days one week and three every other week.

Example:

- Monday – Non-fasting
- Tuesday – Non-fasting
- Wednesday – Fasting
- Thursday – Non-fasting
- Friday – Non-fasting
- Saturday–Fasting
- Sunday – Non-fasting
- Monday – Non-fasting
- Tuesday – Fasting
- Wednesday – Non-fasting
- Thursday – Non-fasting
- Friday– Fasting
- Saturday – Non-fasting
- Sunday – Non-fasting

The Eat Stop Eat plan is generally one where fasting days involve complete abstinence from food and only allow zero-calorie beverages. However, to ease you into this fasting method, you can try restricting calories on fasting days until you build up to whole-day fasts.

CHOOSE YOUR DAY

The Choose Your Day method is an entirely flexible intermittent fasting plan. It can be a combination of several of the above plans. The name says it all. You choose the days on which you want to fast and you can choose between the 16:8 method, a calorie restriction like the Fast 800 and original 5:2 methods, or whole-day complete fasts on your fasting days. You can fast on set days per week or choose your fasting days according to your preference and what is happening in your life at the time. The only requirement, if restricting calories or performing whole-day fasts, is that there is at least one non-fasting day between fasting days.

THE WARRIOR DIET

The name "Warrior Diet" probably brings images of soldiers and battles from times gone by to mind. Those images are quite correct. This intermittent fasting method was developed by a former member of Israel's Special Forces, Ori Hofmekler. When he left the services, he turned his attention to nutrition and fitness. The idea of the Warrior Diet is to mimic the eating patterns ancient warriors used to follow centuries ago. It is historically believed these warriors would not eat very much during the day, but would eat, or rather feast, at night.

The idea is to fast, or eat extremely little, for twenty hours of the day and then eat as much as you like in a four-hour window at the end of the day. Ori encourages eating small amounts of hard-boiled eggs, dairy, and raw vegetables and fruits, and drinking lots of water during those 20 hours. Since we've already discussed not eating too close to bedtime, it's a good idea to schedule your end-of-the-day eating window a few hours before you go to bed.

While you can technically eat whatever you like during your feasting window, it's better to make healthy food choices. Fasting brings with it numerous benefits, but those benefits won't be felt if you're filling up on unhealthy foods. Instead, choose foods that are as natural as possible to ensure that your body receives all of the nutrients it need.

The Warrior Diet is broken up into a three-week, phased schedule, which we will get into in a moment. However, it's vitally important to understand that while the word "feasting" is used when speaking about the Warrior Diet, it's not encouraging you to binge. You have a four-hour window in which to eat. Try spreading your food consumption over that whole period and keep it to a sensible amount. If you dive right in and just start eating everything in sight without pacing yourself, you could end up developing an unhealthy binge-eating relationship with food and that's certainly not what the diet is about.

When feasting, eat a sensible portion of food followed by a 20-minute wait period. This waiting period allows your body and brain to respond to signals of satiety which will tell you if you are full. If you are still hungry after that 20-

minute period, eat another portion of the same food and wait again. This eat-wait-eat cycle will help prevent binge eating.

Week 1: The Detox Phase

This phase of the diet focuses on clearing your body of toxins. You could probably see it as a mild form of "shock treatment," because you're going to be removing animal proteins and wheat from your diet.

- During the 20 hours of under-eating, consume small amounts of clear broth, vegetable juices, dairy, raw vegetables and fruit, and hard-boiled eggs.
- During the feasting window, you should fill up on salad drizzled with a vinaigrette (or oil and vinegar dressing), wheat-free whole grains, plant proteins such as beans and tofu, cooked vegetables, and a little bit of cheese.
- During the day, you can drink water, coffee, tea, and small amounts of milk, but make sure you drink lots of water.

Week 2: The High-Fat Phase

- During the 20 hours of under-eating, consume small amounts of clear broth, vegetable juices, dairy, raw vegetables and fruit, and hard-boiled eggs.

- During the feasting window, you should fill up on a salad drizzled with vinaigrette, lean animal proteins, a minimum of one handful of nuts, and cooked, non-starchy vegetables.
- Starches and grains are cut out of your diet during this phase.

Week 3: The Maintenance Phase

This phase of the diet can be continued indefinitely. It's simply the Warrior Diet's 20:4 schedule with cycling between high-carb and low-carb days. You should alternate one to two days of high carb with one to two days of low carb.

- Fill up on salad and vinaigrette, lean protein, cooked vegetables (especially starchy ones), and carbohydrates such as pasta, corn, or grains on high-carb days.
- Fill up on salad and vinaigrette, between eight and sixteen ounces of lean animal protein, and cooked, non-starchy vegetables on low-carb days.

OMAD

The abbreviation OMAD stands for "One Meal a Day". You guessed it; during this intermittent fasting method, you'll be eating only one meal each day. How is OMAD different from the Warrior Diet? Instead of giving yourself four hours in which to feast on lots of food, with OMAD you only have one hour to eat one meal. You are essentially fasting for 23 hours per day and eating during a one-hour window.

As with the Warrior Diet, OMAD presents the risk of falling into a binge eating pattern and an unhealthy relationship with food. While you are eating only one meal per day; you can spread that meal out over an hour. This will help you apply the eat-wait-eat concept we explained under the Warrior Diet, where you eat a sensible portion and wait 20 minutes before eating a second helping if you're still hungry.

OMAD doesn't dictate what you should be eating or even when you should eat your one meal for the day. The sole requirement is that you eat only once a day within a one-hour window. However, that being said, it's not a good idea to fill up on calorie-dense processed foods that offer you little to no nutrition. You should be focusing on lean animal proteins, fresh and cooked vegetables, fresh fruit, nuts, whole grains, and healthy fats. When possible, stay away from processed meals.

THE BOTTOM LINE

We've gone through the various intermittent fasting plans so that you can choose the one that works best for you. To find the fasting rhythm that works best for you, you may need to experiment a bit.

You should also not take these methods as set in stone. Why? In the next chapter we're going to explore how fasting affects women differently from men and how to overcome the associated challenges women face. We're also going to take a look at why a healthy diet and regular exercise are imperative for your overall health.

4

WOMEN AND FASTING, DIET, AND EXERCISE

Intermittent fasting cannot work health and weight loss miracles on its own. You need to incorporate a healthy, balanced diet and regular exercise into your lifestyle as well. We're going to tell you how fasting affects women and why, as well as the importance of a healthy diet and exercise to achieve your health and weight loss goals.

WOMEN: THE FASTING DIFFERENCE

Women tend to fare better on shorter fasting periods, while men seem to handle longer fasting periods more easily. Why is that? Why can men adapt to the fasting lifestyle easier than women? It doesn't seem fair, does it? There are actually very good biological reasons for women facing an increased challenge when it comes to intermittent fasting. Hold onto your seats and we'll explain it all to you.

You may have heard criticism about intermittent fasting. Some claims include that it causes your hormones to go out of whack, and it will interfere with your thyroid. It may be tempting to listen to these nay-sayers and shy away from the fasting lifestyle, however, please read the following section on the effects of intermittent fasting on women to enable you make an informed choice.

Hunger Hormones

Some of the major hormones that control hunger and how satisfied you feel after a meal include insulin, ghrelin, and leptin. Both men and women deal with these hormones in response to fasting, but women are more sensitive to them.

This is because women have a built-in survival mechanism. After all, women are the ones who ensure the survival of the species and their bodies are programmed to make that happen. You can keep a population going with fewer men as opposed to women but not the other way around. So, evolution has cleverly designed women's bodies to be geared toward surviving, more so than men. That means their bodies essentially overreact when it perceives a shortage of food.

Women experience a more dramatic drop in leptin, the hormone that tells you you're satisfied. This increases the hormones that make you feel hungry in the first place and therefore women get hungrier than men when fasting. Despite the fact that you know you're not in the middle of a famine, your body doesn't make that distinction, so it tries to make you find food and eat.

Reproductive Hormones

It's not only your feeling of hunger that is affected when your body perceives a food shortage. A chain reaction happens. Your hunger hormones kick into overdrive while your reproductive hormones go on a go-slow. Your body is saying, "Hang on, there isn't enough food to keep me going, so how am I going to bring a healthy baby to full term?" In more extreme cases, this perception of a less than optimal environment for having a baby can lead to irregular menstruation or a lack of it altogether.

Thyroid

It's true that your thyroid is influenced by fasting, but it's not as bad as anti-fasting advocates make it out to be. While you're fasting, your thyroid will slow down, but the same thing happens in between meals anyway. So, what happens with your thyroid while you're fasting?

Just like your reproductive hormones are influenced by your hunger hormones, they also have an effect on your thyroid. There are three important hormones when it comes to your thyroid. They are T3, T4, and TSH. The active thyroid hormone that is present in your body at any given point in time is T3. T4 is responsible for the future production of thyroid hormone, T3. TSH is the thyroid-stimulating hormone, which is what prompts the production of T4. The only thyroid hormone that is actually affected by fasting is T3, the active thyroid hormone in your body at this precise moment. Fasting doesn't have an impact on T4 and it doesn't really affect TSH much either.

If you're still worried about how fasting may be affecting your thyroid activity, there is one simple sign to look out for. Are you feeling cold all the time? If you are constantly feeling cold, not only when you are fasting but during your eating window as well, it may indicate a slowing of your thyroid. The emphasis is on the word "may". Being cold all the time doesn't necessarily mean your thyroid is slowing down, but if you're concerned, you should visit your doctor for a check-up and blood tests. That way you'll be able to find out if it's really your thyroid or if there is another reason for feeling cold all the time.

How to Fast as a Woman

It can be worrisome to know that fasting affects your hormones and you may even be reconsidering whether you want to fast or not. Don't let this information discourage you. There are ways around these challenges. Here are some recommendations.

Are you feeling super hungry, like your hunger is unbearable and over-the-top? Break your fast and pick up your fasting plan again tomorrow. By listening to your body, you can pick up on cues telling you that your hormones are at risk of being impacted more than you want them to be.

Doesn't breaking your fast go against the grain of living the fasting lifestyle? No, not at all. It's better for women to fast a few days a week as opposed to fasting every single day. Women, and their hormones, will fare much better fasting a maximum of three to four days per week instead of trying to go all out every day of the week. This is one reason the 5:2 fasting method is voted as one of the best intermittent fasting methods for women. If two days a week seems too little; you can always increase that to three or four.

Another option would be to try fasting for shorter periods of time. Instead of trying to fast for extended periods of time, start off with 12 or 14 hours. Actually, just as women do well on the 5:2 or Choose Your Day fasting methods where they are only fasting a couple of days per week, they also do much better on shorter fasting periods if they do want to try fasting more often than just a few days a week.

The key to successfully fasting as a woman is to listen to your body. We cannot say this enough. Your body will tell you when it's not happy with what you are doing. Take a break from fasting if you feel that your hormones are out of kilter and making you feel cold, unwell, or moody.

Fasting Mistakes

We've already established that women are much more sensitive to hunger hormones than men. That's why their bodies have a stronger reaction and their hormones end up all over the place, but that's not all. Many women try to do far too much. They try to fast too long or too often. They try to combine intermittent fasting with a severe calorie restriction to slim down faster. They may try hard diets like keto. They may also try to ramp up their exercise by packing in tons of cardio and heavy resistance training.

Fasting is already going to place stress on your body until it learns to adapt to your new lifestyle. You really don't need to push it to its limit by trying to do too much all at once. Your body isn't going to know what hit it and it's going to go crazy trying to compensate for what it perceives as a lack of food, calories, and nutrition, in combination with overexertion.

Again, take it easy and take it slowly. Intermittent fasting is already a big lifestyle change to adapt to. Listen to your body. Let's say it again: listen to your body.

Eat enough calories. If you want to create a calorie deficit, make it an extremely modest one. Don't try to slash your intake by 1,000 calories per day because you've heard that will produce a two-pound weight loss per week.

Make sure you are getting enough nutrition by eating a balanced diet that isn't swayed to an extreme by cutting out food groups. Eat healthy, whole foods to ensure you're getting in all your vitamins and minerals.

Don't try to sweat it out on the treadmill every day until your legs feel like they're not going to carry you to the shower. In fact, you should probably bring any cardio you're already doing down a notch.

Try light strength training with bodyweight exercises like lunges and squats. Fit in gentle cardio like walking that will get you moving but not overtax your body. Maintain your range of motion and flexibility with some gentle yoga.

THE IMPORTANCE OF A HEALTHY DIET AND EXERCISE

It can be tempting to indulge on your non-fasting days. This is a psychological hurdle to overcome. Overeating or following a poor diet on non-fasting days isn't justified by fasting. This mindset opens the door to developing a dysfunctional relationship with food and disordered eating habits.

Aim for maintaining a healthy diet and eating mindfully on non-fasting days, otherwise you can find yourself back where you started, or worse, you could end up overeating and gaining weight instead of losing it. If you're following a plan like the Fast 800 and reach stage two or stage three, allowing your diet to fall by the wayside may see you having to start from the beginning again. Doing this would constitute yo-yo dieting, which isn't healthy and could lead to weight loss difficulties every time you try to drop the weight.

Just like diet, exercise is a crucial part of a holistically healthy lifestyle, transforming your body and health and allowing you to maintain a healthy weight. Including exercise in your fasting lifestyle amplifies the health benefits associated with fasting. Other benefits of daily exercise include:

- Weight loss and weight maintenance following weight loss
- Improved mobility and flexibility
- Better respiratory capacity and health
- More energy
- Stress relief
- Better mood, due to the release of natural feel-good hormones
- Improved mental health
- Better sleep quality
- Increased muscle and bone strength
- Improved balance and lower risk of falling

While regular exercise doesn't provide health benefits in exactly the same way as intermittent fasting, many of the same benefits are provided, such as:

- Healthier heart
- Lowered blood pressure
- Boosting metabolism
- Insulin and blood sugar regulation
- Reduced risk of various cancers

EXERCISING WHILE PRACTICING INTERMITTENT FASTING

You can and should exercise while following an intermittent fasting plan. However, there is a right and wrong way to go about it safely. Intermittent fasting involves either complete abstinence from food or a considerable restriction of your calorie intake. This will have an influence on your energy levels, at least in the beginning. Going too hard on exercise while your body adjusts to your new fasting lifestyle could see you give up on both healthy lifestyle choices by over-taxing your body. Here is how to safely exercise while practicing intermittent fasting.

Take It Easy

Walking and intermittent fasting are the ultimate weight loss power couple. They go hand in hand so perfectly that they seem like the proverbial "match made in heaven," and there are three prime reasons for this.

Intermittent fasting is a healthy, safe, and effective lifestyle choice to help lose unwanted pounds and keep them off. It can be practiced indefinitely, which is why it's not a diet in the typical sense of the word. It becomes a part of your life, not a temporary weight loss fix. It is a lifestyle, just like engaging in regular exercise is a healthy lifestyle habit.

Walking is an underrated, yet highly effective, form of exercise that really works for weight loss and overall health. It is accessible to almost everyone, so few have an excuse not to get their daily dose of exercise. You can do it almost any time and anywhere.

Running is often considered the ultimate cardiovascular workout. What nobody tells you is that walking has similar heart health benefits as running. In addition to being a cardiovascular workout, walking is low impact and won't put stress on your joints and bones. It is the perfect exercise for newcomers to the world of a healthy lifestyle through the inclusion of regular exercise.

Finally, we have to consider the effect fasting can have on your energy. The initial stages of adjusting to intermittent fasting can make intense exercise draining. Trying to exercise when your body feels fatigued because it's not used to periods of fasting can set you up for exercise failure. Starting off with easy, gentle exercise is a sure-fire way to adopting a healthy lifestyle and maintaining it in the long term.

Timing Is Everything

Are you the kind of person who performs physical activity well on an empty stomach, or are you better suited to getting physical after a good meal? When it comes to incorporating walking into your intermittent fasting lifestyle, this is a crucial question to answer.

- If exercising on an empty stomach gives you a boost of energy, go ahead and get your walk in before your eating window begins.
- If you feel better and more energized after a meal and want to use post-workout nutrition to combat the potential after-exercise energy drop, go for your walk during your eating window.
- If taking a walk during your eating window isn't possible and you don't like to do exercise on an empty stomach, get your walking exercise in shortly after your last meal.

Walking at the right time for your personal preference and fasting schedule is vital for motivation and for maintaining a regular exercise regime.

Tip: It has been suggested that exercising while in a fasted state has the potential to increase the fat burn from physical activity. However, if exercising in a fasted state isn't for you, don't try to force it upon your body. Intermittent fasting and walking will get you to your goal, irrespective of the timing, as long as you do both things safely and comfortably.

HEALTHY DIET, HEALTHY BODY

Intermittent fasting is a fantastic lifestyle choice to help you transform your body and your life through weight loss and improved health. However, fasting can't do it all alone. Though intermittent fasting focus on when you eat, what you eat can have a significant impact on your ability to burn fat.

It cannot be stressed enough that eating a healthy diet during your eating window or on non-fasting days is essential for intermittent fasting to work. Cycling between fasting and eating won't have any effect if you are eating the wrong foods or eating too much when you break your fast. Enjoying healthy, nutritious foods in between fasting periods will also help you to feel more satisfied and less hungry with fewer cravings.

The Mediterranean Diet

The Mediterranean diet, often known as the Med diet, is based on the eating habits of people living in the Mediterranean Sea region in the 1960s. To this day, it remains one of the healthiest diets worldwide.

The U.S. News and World Report ranks the Mediterranean diet as the best overall diet for the following reasons:

- Best overall diet
- Best plant-based diet
- Best heart-healthy diet
- Best diabetes diet
- Best diet for healthy eating
- Easiest diet to follow

These rankings are determined by a panel of experts consisting of nutritionists, dieticians, diabetes and heart disease specialists, and other experts in medical fields pertaining to diet and nutrition.

The joy of the Mediterranean diet is that it isn't as strict as some other diets and there are no food groups that are excluded or drastically reduced. The Med diet doesn't take inspiration from just one country or culture. The Mediterranean Sea is bordered by a number of countries. Instead, the diet draws on the diet, flavors, and foods grown in different regions of several countries. Due to this regional and cultural variety, the Mediterranean diet never gets boring and can be adapted based on the seasonal availability of fruits and vegetables.

One of the most attractive aspects of the Med diet is how easy it is to follow. Simply move away from processed foods and focus on fresh, whole foods, lean meats and seafood, and whole grains. That's it – it really is that simple and easy. Because it's so straightforward, the Mediterranean diet is likely to deliver long-term success, making a healthy lifestyle a breeze.

Mediterranean Diet Breakdown

A focus on daily activity is at the heart of the Mediterranean diet. It need not be an intense or rigorous activity; you just need to get your body moving every day. This makes walking a perfect match for the Med diet's daily physical activity requirement.

The basis of every meal in the Mediterranean diet is whole grains and fresh or cooked vegetables – lots of them. Ensure that you opt for whole grains such as brown rice, whole wheat pasta, and oatmeal. Refined grains make up the bulk of grains consumed in a typical Western diet, but they aren't nearly as healthy as whole grains. When it comes to vegetables and fruit, fresh is best and you are encouraged to eat a wide variety, ensuring that your body gets all the vital nutrients it needs.

Only a small portion of a meal is made up of seafood, lean meat, or poultry. Think of these portions as side servings instead of being the bulk of the meal. The focus is placed on seafood over poultry or red meat. That's not to say you should only eat fish and seafood. Moderate amounts of poultry are good for you, but red meat should be kept to no more than once a week. On the Med diet, a basic rule of thumb is to limit red meat consumption to 17-18 ounces (500g) each month.

Emphasis is placed on home-cooked meals. The Mediterranean diet encourages you to move away from processed foods packed with additives, preservatives, and other potentially harmful ingredients. You should also choose sustainably sourced, free-range, and hormone- and antibiotic-free meat, seafood, poultry, and dairy. The idea is to focus on foods that are natural and not overly processed, but that doesn't mean you can't use some canned, bottled, or packaged foods; just try to keep them to a minimum.

Fats are encouraged on the Mediterranean diet. Yes, you read that correctly. As part of a healthy diet, fat plays a crucial role in the absorption of fat-soluble vitamins, which can only be efficiently digested if they are present in fat.

However, not all fat is created equal. There are good fats, namely unsaturated fats, and there are bad fats, namely man-made trans fats. The fats included in the Mediterranean diet are healthy, unsaturated fats such as olive oil. Olive oil is an essential component of the Mediterranean diet, and many followers will use it on their bread instead of butter and as a salad dressing.

Speaking of fat; on the Med diet, low-fat foods are not your friends. Why? Low-fat foods and foods otherwise labeled 'diet' or 'light' are generally highly processed and trick you into opting for them over less processed, full-fat foods with the lure of a lower calorie count.

While fat is encouraged, sugar is not. Whenever possible, opt for unsweetened foods, such as unsweetened yogurt. It's also a good idea to attempt to limit how much sugar you consume in your diet, such as in your coffee and tea, or over your breakfast cereal. Cutting back on sugar also means cutting back on the sweet stuff like chocolate, cakes, sweets, etc. You are encouraged to add a bit of natural sweetness to your life instead by enjoying fresh or cooked fruit with no added sugar.

Looking at the macronutrients, or macros, of the Mediterranean diet, it is a moderate carb and protein diet with a higher healthy fat intake than a regular Western healthy balanced diet. You're looking at approximately:

- 40% carbohydrates
- 20-25% protein
- 35-40% fat

Now that you know what you should eat, let's look at how much of it you should be eating per day or week.

- Lots of fresh or cooked vegetables daily, as much as you want
- Whole grains form part of almost every meal
- 2-3 servings of fruit per day
- 1-3 servings of legumes, beans, nuts, and seeds per day
- 0-2 servings of seafood and fish, poultry, and eggs per day
- 1-2 servings of full-fat dairy per day
- Consumption of healthy fats like olive oil is encouraged
- Red meat makes an occasional appearance, but isn't high on the priority list

- Junk food and sweets are to be consumed as a very occasional treat

How Does the Mediterranean Diet Encourage Weight Loss?

How does the Mediterranean diet help you lose weight, given that it is built on whole grains and many weight loss regimes encourage limiting carbs? The type of carbohydrates consumed on the Mediterranean diet is key to weight loss success.

The carbohydrates that come from whole grains are complex, whereas the carbs from refined grains, like white flour, are simple. Simple carbs are quick and easy to break down into sugars and digest, flooding your body with near-instant energy in one go. You experience a sudden blood sugar spike and very soon, your body removes all that sugar from your blood and your energy drops. This leaves you hungry and craving another dose of high-energy, easy-to-digest carbs.

Complex carbohydrates, on the other hand, take longer to digest, offering your body near-constant, slow-release energy as the food is digested. This serves to keep you feeling satisfied longer, staving off hunger and cravings for calorie-rich, low-nutrient foods. Not only does this prevent snacking and feeling hungry shortly after a meal, but you are also likely to naturally eat fewer calories.

THE BOTTOM LINE

Women face increased challenges when taking up the fasting lifestyle and you now have a better understanding of what those challenges are and how to deal with them.

Another crucial aspect to successfully transforming your life through practicing intermittent fasting is to develop a fasting lifestyle, exercise habits, and an overall healthy living mindset. We're going to get into that in the next chapter to help you to build the mentality necessary to stick to your new fasting schedule and healthy lifestyle changes.

5

INTERMITTENT FASTING: HOW TO START

Yes, intermittent fasting is a healthy lifestyle choice and a powerful tool for self-transformation, but it's not something you can just dive into head first without knowing how to start. There may be psychological barriers in place that could stop you from fasting with success and if there are, they must be removed before you can start.

There is a right way and a wrong way to start fasting and to break a fast. There are some things to be aware of before you start so they don't catch you by surprise. Preparing for an intermittent fasting lifestyle is about more than just deciding to skip a few meals. It takes knowledge to effectively make the transition to increase your success rate.

INTERMITTENT FASTING MINDSET

Any substantial lifestyle change starts with one thing: your mindset. You cannot effect change if your head isn't in the game. It's not good enough to just want to change: you also have to change how you think about things. Trying to make external changes while maintaining old thought patterns will only make the challenge of changing more difficult. That being said, what are the mental barriers that may prevent you from succeeding at intermittent fasting, and how do you overcome them?

It's a Lifestyle

We've said it before, and it cannot be said enough, but let's look at a more in-depth explanation of why changing the way you think about intermittent fasting as a lifestyle instead of a diet is vital for success. Intermittent fasting often gets labeled as a diet, but that does it no justice.

The very first mental shift you need to make is to see intermittent fasting as a long-term lifestyle, and not just a short-term fix for weight loss. Changing your perspective and how you label fasting will change how you feel while fasting. It will also increase your resolve in the early days when your body is still adjusting to the new eating pattern.

In our modern age, the word "diet" has taken on a negative meaning. What do you think of when you hear it? Chances are, the thoughts revolve around self-deprivation and unpleasant feelings. You may also conjure up images of all the fat-free, light, and diet items on store shelves. You are already building up a mental scenario of a diet being an unpleasant experience. You may also be experiencing feelings of dread and thinking about how long you'll have to endure the unpleasant business of dieting.

Typical dieting is also done for short periods, which, coincidentally, is one of the reasons it doesn't work. Diets are associated with drastic measures taken to achieve drastic results. After all, we live in an instant gratification world and we want what we want and we want it right now, so the sooner you lose weight, the better, right? Not quite.

The journey of healthy and sustainable weight loss taken to transform your body and health teaches you about yourself. It allows you to make a permanent change for lasting health and happiness. You don't want to go on a diet. You want to make a healthy lifestyle change for long-term success, and not just temporary satisfaction. Thinking about intermittent fasting as a diet may be fostering a negative attitude before you have even tried fasting. When you see things in a negative way, your perception of them becomes negative by default.

Your mind will actively seek out the negatives while you're trying to fast and it will do its best to convince you to give up.

Lifestyle changes are typically viewed in a more positive light than dieting. Lifestyle changes are associated with long-term success, satisfaction, and achieving truly important goals. Lifestyle changes are also often difficult to make, but when you think about a lifestyle change that will help you reach your goals, you feel more positive about it. Viewing something in a positive way helps your mind to seek out the positives, strengthen your resolve, and make even difficult aspects seem easier.

Getting into the fasting lifestyle isn't easy. You have to go against long-standing habits, overhaul your lifestyle, and give your body time to adjust. However, once your body does adjust, fasting becomes as easy as following your previous lifestyle. Before you start a fasting lifestyle, you need to change your attitude toward it. Build up a positive mental scenario. Focus on the positive, long-term lifestyle change. It's not just for now; it's for your future happiness. Keep your eyes on the prizes that are your weight loss and your health goals.

Core Beliefs, Food Rules, and Internal Dialogue

Your beliefs about food shape the way you think about it, how you interact with it, what rules you have about it, and how you speak to yourself about it. Once you've acknowledged that intermittent fasting is a lifestyle, it's time to change what you believe about food and eating.

Core Beliefs

Core beliefs shape how you perceive the world, not only how you view food. They are ingrained so deeply that you may not even realize you have them. These core beliefs develop in childhood and sometimes in adulthood in response to powerful experiences. If you have rigid core beliefs about food that are not factually correct, but rather come from a place of subjectivity, they may be standing in the way of success.

Changing core beliefs can be challenging, but it isn't impossible. These are beliefs you hold about anything and everything that were passed down to you by your parents, society, and from personal experience. Many times, core beliefs are not necessarily based on fact, but rather on an opinion or an accepted view. Looking at the facts can help you change your beliefs and mold them into beliefs that will help you to reach your weight loss and health goals.

Changing Core Beliefs

Core beliefs vary from person to person. It will take time and introspection to identify which core beliefs need changing. Here are some examples of core beliefs and how to change them to give you an idea of what to look for and how to challenge them.

CORE BELIEF: CHANGE

Core Belief	Change
You may believe that you don't deserve happiness, health, and weight loss due to self-deprecation.	Challenge self-deprecation to establish your self-worth and begin believing that you deserve health, happiness, and weight loss.
You may believe that fasting equates to self-starvation and is harmful, not healthy.	Look at the facts and acknowledge that fasting isn't starving yourself and that research shows it's a healthy lifestyle.
You may believe that if something takes a lot of effort and happens slowly instead of being easy and quick, you can't do it.	Develop your self-worth to begin believing that you are worth the effort it takes and that you can accomplish anything you set your mind to, even if it doesn't happen instantly.
You may associate fasting solely with religious practices and penance.	Challenge this belief and realize the incredible health benefits that intermittent fasting can provide.

These examples aren't the only potential core beliefs that could be barriers to intermittent fasting success. You may or may not have some of these beliefs. Take the time to really think about intermittent fasting and observe your thoughts. Pick out the thoughts that convey negativity and begin to challenge them and, in so doing, change your core beliefs over time.

Food Rules

Food rules, like core beliefs, shape your attitude toward food and eating and they are also often based on subjective opinion, rather than hard facts. Your core beliefs are often where food rules come from. Your personal food rules may be influenced by teachings from your parents, habits and beliefs held by your peers, or by society as a whole, or the seed may have been planted by media sources such as social media and magazines. Irrespective of where your food rules come from or why you have them, it's important to determine what they are and whether they are helpful or harmful to your intermittent fasting goals.

Food rules are not just about the actual food you eat. They also involve eating habits. For instance, a low-carb dieter can have the core belief that carbs are bad. They have the food rule of eating only the lowest-carb foods available. A food rule like this doesn't stem from fact, because carbohydrates, in themselves, are not bad and actually form a vital part of a healthy diet. However, the rule is based on what they have been told and perhaps their own personal experience with carbs.

The take-home message is that food rules need to be examined and changed, depending on whether they help you or stand in your way.

Changing Food Rules

There are some common food rules that we can look at as examples to help you get started on determining your own food rules and changing the ones that prevent you from fasting successfully.

Core Belief and Corresponding Food Rule	Change
Core belief: Breakfast is the most important meal of the day. **Food rule:** Always eat breakfast shortly after getting up in the morning.	Look at the facts and research that suggest the contrary. Recognize the food rule isn't helpful and let it go.
Core belief: You must do what others are doing to fit in. **Food rule:** Always eat when others eat.	Realize that your social circle already accepts you and that always eating when others eat won't make you an outcast in social settings.
Core belief: Refusing something is impolite or very rude. **Food rule:** Always accept and eat food when it is offered.	Realize that a polite refusal isn't the height of rudeness and that accepting food you don't necessarily want to eat may be harmful.

Internal Dialogue

Your internal dialogue refers to how you speak to yourself. It is self-talk and it can be very persuasive. The problem is that self-talk is influenced by core beliefs and food rules that aren't necessarily correct. By affecting how you see and feel about yourself, self-talk has the potential to make or break your happiness.

Your internal dialogue is a powerful tool to use when you are trying to challenge and change unhelpful beliefs, thoughts, and behaviors, so it's important to pay attention to what that little voice inside your head is telling you. If you let it rule the roost, because you are not paying attention to how it is influencing you, you could be stuck in habits and beliefs that stand in your way of transforming your body and your life.

Let's take a closer look at how core beliefs influence internal dialogue and ultimately, your behavior.

You may hold the core belief that you aren't capable of achieving your dreams. This core belief translates into internal dialogue when you tell yourself that intermittent fasting will be too hard and you aren't capable of achieving it. This belief and internal dialogue is self-deprecating and sucks all the motivation and determination out of you. It may even stop you from attempting intermittent fasting.

It is important to identify core beliefs and pay attention to what your self-talk is saying to you. Don't let any self-talk go unchallenged. Pick out the unhelpful internal dialogue, challenge it by turning it into something positive, and repeat the process over and over. Self-talk occurs often and it usually repeats itself like a broken record. Challenging your internal dialogue aids in challenging and changing your core beliefs. The results will not be instantaneous, but they will be achieved with consistency and effort.

Another trick you can try is developing personal affirmations to use as a mantra during the day. These are short positive phrases like "I'm making a positive lifestyle change for better health." or "I can and will reach my healthy weight.". Affirmations are great for motivating yourself when you feel your motivation wavers.

Emotional Eating

There are several misconceptions about emotional eating that allow it to get swept under the rug and largely be ignored. People may think that unless they are binging on vast amounts of high-calorie junk food, they aren't eating for emotional reasons. They may think that emotional eating is exclusively a female problem and that men don't eat to satisfy emotions. People may not even realize they are emotional eaters, because it has become such a habit that they don't even think about why or what they are eating.

Emotional eating may be a serious emotional and psychological obstacle standing in the way of successful intermittent fasting. If you're aware that you're an emotional eater, it's time to take charge and start changing how you deal with emotions.

If you're unsure whether or not you're an emotional eater, ask yourself some simple questions to help figure it out:

- Do you feel powerless to control yourself around food?
- Do you eat when you aren't actually hungry?
- Do you overeat until you're bursting at the seams?
- Do you reach for food in response to negative emotions as a means to soothe and calm yourself?
- Do you reward yourself for achievement by grabbing something to eat or drink?

- Do you find that you eat more when you are feeling stressed?
- Do you see food as a kind of friend or security blanket that makes you feel safe?

These questions aren't a definitive indication of emotional eating, but they do offer a chance to really think about your eating habits and how you view food. Emotional eating is a big hurdle to get over if you want to practice intermittent fasting. During your fasting period, you cannot simply reach for a snack whenever your emotions tell you that you need one to deal with stress, negative emotions, boredom, etc. You have to find a healthier alternative or coping strategy to replace eating so that your emotions and linked eating habits don't derail your fasting efforts.

What Is the Trigger?

Before you can find a suitable alternative or coping strategy, you need to identify what is triggering your emotional eating. While everyone's triggers are unique, the following are some frequent causes:

- Emotions that are unpleasant and difficult to deal with
- Stress
- Associating food with reward, often learned as a child by being rewarded with sweets for achievements or good behavior

- Social anxiety and nervousness around others in social settings
- Being encouraged to eat, even if you don't want to, and feeling bad or guilty if you refuse
- Boredom
- Feelings of emptiness

Once you've identified out what's causing your emotional eating, it's time to come up with a solution that doesn't involve food. Using food to placate negative emotions requires facing those emotions and dealing with them instead of trying to bury them with food. There is always a better, healthier coping option for any situation in which your emotions lead you to food. Healthy coping mechanisms look different for different women. Some may find it useful to use a breathing exercise to bring their emotions under control. Others may find journaling helpful. It's critical to have a coping strategy that works for you.

HOW TO START FASTING

You've removed potential emotional and psychological barriers that could be blocking your path to intermittent fasting and you're ready to start, but how do you go about doing that?

First and foremost, consult your doctor. We said it in the first chapter and we're saying it again here. Always ensure you consult your family physician to get the all-clear before you embark upon any lifestyle changes that can affect your health and well-being.

The next thing you need to do is to make sure you are already following a healthy diet. Trying to fast and adopt a healthy diet, which may be completely different to your current diet at the same time, puts you under too much pressure mentally, emotionally, and physically. You are likely to increase your chances of failing or giving up if you try to do too much all at once. When you've been following a healthy diet for a few weeks and your body has adjusted to your new diet, then you can start your fasting program.

Beginner Plan: Easing into Intermittent Fasting

Before Beginning Fasting

Don't try to go all-in right away with long fasting periods, especially if you've never fasted before. It will be an unpleasant experience for your body, may make it more difficult to stick to your fasting period. Gradually introduce fasting by following these tips:

- If you're a post-dinner snacker, give up your evening snacking habit.
- Slowly phase out daytime snacking between meals. You don't have to cut all snacks out to begin with. Cut them out one at a time. Once you're used to not having a morning snack, cut out your afternoon snack as well.

When Beginning Fasting

- Start overnight fasting by fasting for 12 hours from the moment you take your last dinner bite.
- Start with a shorter fasting period and gradually increase the length of your fasting period as your body adjusts. Once you're accustomed to a 12-hour fast, bump it up to 13 hours, and so on.
- If you do decide to start with a longer fasting period of up to 16 hours, don't beat yourself up if the hunger pangs overwhelm you and you have to break your fast early. Often a small, low-calorie snack can help, but it's important to know what counts. We will get into that later in this chapter.
- If your goal is to do whole-day, strict fasts, start by lowering your calorie intake on your intended fast days. As your body adjusts to fewer calories on fasting days, lower your calorie intake further until you can comfortably fast for a whole day.

Important note: It is vital to listen to your body, whether you are still easing into fasting or have become accustomed to the intermittent fasting lifestyle. If you feel unwell at any time during your fasting period or on your fasting day, break your fast or don't fast. It's better to break your fast early or skip a fasting day than to put your health at risk. Remember, you can always give it another go tomorrow.

What to Expect When Starting Out

Intermittent fasting is a safe, healthy, and effective lifestyle that will help you to shed unwanted pounds and maintain a healthy weight. We covered the various popular intermittent fasting plans and told you how to get started, but what can you expect during your initial adjustment period?

Important note: Starting out on the fasting lifestyle isn't a walk in the park. Your body has to adjust to a whole new lifestyle and there are some things you will experience during this time. Fortunately, these effects are just temporary and will decrease away as your body gets adjusted to intermittent fasting. When faced with challenges, keep reminding yourself of your long-term body and health transformation goals and know that any initial challenges won't last forever.

Hunger

When you get started with intermittent fasting, hunger is an inevitable part of the adaptation process. Hunger will be most intense during the first few days as your body learns to use fat as energy in the absence of sugars. Ghrelin will also still be released according to your old eating schedule. Hunger pangs will subside as your body gets used to your new lifestyle.

Important note: If hunger becomes so strong that it interferes with your ability to function normally, it's best to eat something and rethink the length of your fasting period.

Fasting isn't about self-starvation, so allow your body adequate time to adjust at its own pace, instead of trying to force it to adapt faster, as this is key to success.

Energy Fluctuations

Fatigue is a normal part of adjusting to the intermittent fasting lifestyle. When your body enters a fasted state, you enter the metabolic state of ketosis where your body burns fat for fuel. It is a temporary physical adjustment and your energy levels will increase again once you get used to using fat for energy during your fasting periods.

Mood Fluctuations

Hunger and fatigue influence your mood. Think about the term "hangry". It's made from the words hungry and angry. Hunger tends to make you cranky and fatigue compounds the feeling of grumpiness. Your mood will improve as your body becomes accustomed to using fat for fuel and your hunger pangs subside.

Social Questioning

Intermittent fasting is plagued by myths and misconceptions. Not everybody will understand your choice, what intermittent fasting is, and how it works to improve health and aid weight loss. Fasting is often seen as starving yourself. It is a contradiction of what people are taught about eating regular meals. This makes intermittent fasting confusing to others and you are going to get some questions and possibly some opposition.

Even friends and family may question or debate your choice to adopt a fasting lifestyle. It's best to use the knowledge you have gained from reading this book to provide sensible and informed answers. You need to be prepared to politely refuse food offerings during your fasting period and request that your choices be respected.

You may even find some friends and family to be unsupportive of your decision. Get support from friends and family who are supportive and avoid getting into arguments with those who don't understand. It's your choice, not theirs, and you will just end up frustrated and angry after an argument that does your mood and mental well-being no good.

Tip: If you don't know anybody in your closer social circles who also practices intermittent fasting, try to make friends with others who live the fasting lifestyle through social media or other forums. This will help to prevent feeling isolated and will offer additional support.

BREAKING YOUR FAST

Breaking your fast may seem like it doesn't need any explanation at all. You can just eat whatever you like and however much you want, right? Not quite. Breaking your fast requires thought and there are some dos and don'ts that will make breaking your fast easy and healthy.

Your First Meal

Your first meal when breaking a short-term fast, or one that lasts up to 24 hours, should include a good mix of healthy fats, protein, and complex carbohydrates. A balanced meal will allow you to refuel your body in a way that makes you feel satisfied and will offer a slow energy release. It will not cause a rapid rise in blood sugar, which is typically followed by a steep drop. Spikes and drops in blood sugar only leave you feeling hungrier and craving high-calorie snacks and foods.

Types of Food to Include

- Eat whole foods that include carbohydrates, protein, and fat, but keep the carbs low to moderate. A rule of thumb would be to build your first meal around vegetables and lean protein. Vegetables offer carbohydrates in low amounts.
- Choose whole grains over processed grains.

What Should You Eat?

- Vegetable soup
- Vegetable juice, as fruit juice contains a lot of natural sugar and could cause a blood sugar spike and consequent crash
- Bone broth

- Vegetables and fruit; try to stick with vegetables, as fruit contains a lot of sugar
- Healthy fats, including olive oil and avocado
- Lean protein, such as poultry or fish

A Note on Portion Size

It may be tempting to pile food onto your plate after a fast. After all, you're hungry. However, fasting isn't a get-out-of-jail-free card that gives you license to eat whatever you want and over-indulge in junk food or high-calorie foods that offer little in the way of nutrition. As we've explained before, to effectively lose weight and improve your health by practicing intermittent fasting, following a healthy, calorie-conscious diet during your eating window is imperative.

It is important you keep portion sizes reasonable. If you eat too much during your first meal, you may be left feeling uncomfortably full and bloated.

Foods to Avoid for Your First Meal

Your body may struggle to handle certain foods as part of your first meal after several hours of fasting. Here's a rundown of what to avoid for your first meal when breaking your fast:

- Alcohol on an empty stomach is never a good idea. You will feel its effects quicker and more powerfully. In addition to that, alcohol sugars don't affect your

blood sugar in the same way as regular sugar and won't provide your body with the necessary energy it needs.
- Eggs
- Nuts, seeds, nut butters
- Dairy products
- Red meat may be difficult to digest right after a fast
- Cruciferous vegetables that have not been cooked. Cruciferous vegetables are those that contain calcium salt and include cauliflower, cabbage, and others
- Sugary beverages

Important note: You don't have to abstain from these foods completely. They should only be avoided as part of your first meal when you break your fast.

TIPS AND TRICKS FOR INTERMITTENT FASTING

Big lifestyle changes can be a challenge, and a little help never goes amiss when dealing with these challenges. Here are some tips and tricks to help make the transition to an intermittent fasting lifestyle a bit easier.

Hot beverages

Hot beverages feel more filling than cold ones. Make sure you don't add your regular milk, cream, or creamer that will break your fast. A natural, non-nutritive sweetener will do the trick instead of sugar.

Don't Feast

We've just told you not to eat too much when you break your fast. Aside from making you feel uncomfortable, and possibly even fatigued, feasting when you break your fast could lead you to develop unhealthy eating patterns like binge eating.

Avoid Unintentionally Breaking Your Fast

It is important to know what you can and cannot drink or eat during your fasting period. You don't want to break your fast unintentionally and miss out on the benefits of fasting. There is a lot of debate around the topic of whether or not you can eat and what you should eat during your fasting period. It's suggested that eating a small, extremely low-carb snack under 50 calories may be alright.

Keep Yourself Busy

Boredom is known to encourage feelings of hunger, cravings, and the desire to snack. These feelings will be intensified during your fasting period and may lead to a preoccupation with food. Keeping yourself busy prevents boredom and those amplified desires to snack and minimize cravings.

Stay Hydrated

Sometimes thirst can mimic hunger. Combining mimicked feelings from thirst and actual hunger intensifies your feelings of being hungry. Hydration is also important for optimal health and has a hand in burning fat, so drink up both while fasting and during your eating window.

Monitor Your Caffeine Intake

As a warm beverage and an appetite suppressant, coffee may seem like the ideal drink during your fasting period. As with everything, enjoy coffee and other caffeinated drinks in moderation (about 4 cups per day is safe for those who aren't particularly sensitive to caffeine), as too much caffeine may cause unpleasant side effects which could make you feel terrible and make sticking to your fasting schedule more difficult.

MYTHS AND FREQUENTLY ASKED QUESTIONS

Intermittent fasting is shrouded in conflicting information and misinformation based on assumptions, rather than facts. People are quick to form subjective, possibly even prejudiced, opinions about the fasting lifestyle, based on very little information or the wrong information.

Word of mouth is said to be one of the best forms of advertising, but it can also give rise to myths and misconceptions. In this section, we are going to dispel those myths and answer questions that may still be lingering, even after having come so far in reading this book.

Busting Myths

Not all of these myths are about intermittent fasting, specifically. Some of them are general diet and eating pattern myths that have no solid base in science. They may be core beliefs or food rules you have based on what you have been taught by society at large. However, they all share one trait, and that is, they are not facts. Let's bust some intermittent fasting myths.

Frequent, Small Meals Increase Metabolism

Originally you were taught to eat three square meals per day with healthy morning and afternoon snacks in between meals. Then came the revelation that you should eat smaller meals more frequently instead of three larger meals. The rationale behind eating smaller, more frequent meals is to keep your metabolism going, like feeding coals into a fire stokes the fire to keep it burning continuously.

The other side to that argument coin is that eating less frequently slows your metabolism down. Hence, the conclusion is that eating more frequently keeps your metabolism from slowing down and also increases it by keeping your body constantly burning calories.

How much scientific evidence is there to prove, beyond a shadow of a doubt, that eating frequent small meals does what it's suggested to do? That's just it, it's only a suggestion. Evidence actually points to breakfast not impacting your metabolism as it was once believed to do. It also only applies to an all-day eating pattern, not to a fasting lifestyle. Eating fewer meals during a typical eating schedule doesn't put your body into a fasted state.

If eating less frequently is your metabolism's kryptonite, why have so many people experienced weight loss success by practicing the fasting lifestyle? If intermittent fasting doesn't work, why is there so much research being done to definitively prove the associated health benefits?

Important note: Each individual is different and unique. We may all have the same organs and general body composition, but there is a lot of variability in how our bodies function. The meal frequency that works best for someone else may not work for you. Intermittent fasting comes in many shapes and forms. Choosing the right plan is imperative for success.

Regular Meals Aid Weight Loss

As we've just explained, eating frequently doesn't magically power up your metabolism, and eating less frequently doesn't suddenly bring it to a grinding halt. If meal frequency doesn't have a major impact on metabolism in a regular eating schedule, why would it play a role in your weight loss journey? Fasting, on the other hand, has proven weight loss benefits once your body enters a fasted state and starts burning fat for fuel.

Skipping Breakfast Leads to Weight Gain and is Unhealthy.

Remember a common core belief and food rule which we mentioned in an earlier chapter about breakfast? That it is the most essential meal of the day? This is another dietary myth that is widely believed, but it has no foundation in science.

In January 2019, Tim Spector, a professor of genetic epidemiology at King's College in London, published new findings. These tradition-shattering research findings have been published in the British Medical Journal and paint an entirely different picture about our ingrained breakfast beliefs with new Australian research. The research shows that breakfast is not the most important meal of the day. There is no evidence to correlate eating breakfast to improved metabolic rate or weight loss. In fact, skipping breakfast may actually help you to lose weight.

Important note: Researchers suggest that despite their findings, the results aren't universal. Each person is different and this individual variability determines whether someone will function better by either eating breakfast or skipping the meal. If you are one of those who finds that you function better by eating breakfast, you can easily adapt your intermittent fasting schedule so your eating window is earlier in the day, allowing you to enjoy a late breakfast and an earlier dinner.

Frequent Meals Keep Hunger at Bay

Like everything else, hunger is an individualistic thing. How often you need to eat depends entirely on your own body, not on recommendations for anyone else. However, as we've said before, fasting changes your eating schedule and your body learns to adapt. It will release ghrelin according to your new eating window, thus decreasing hunger pangs as you get used to intermittent fasting.

Fasting Puts You into Starvation Mode

Fasting is commonly misunderstood to be a form of self-starvation. The idea that you are starving yourself through extreme calorie restriction or prolonged periods of not eating leads to the assumption that your body will go into what is termed "starvation mode". Starvation mode is real and it does exist, but it's more complex and less powerful than you think.

Starvation mode occurs when your body is deprived of the energy and nutrition necessary to function properly. It is crucial to understand that starvation happens over a long period of time – it doesn't just happen after a few hours of fasting. Starvation is accompanied by very serious malnutrition and loss of lean muscle mass. This causes your body to slow your metabolism down to preserve as much energy as it can. Fasting for a few hours, even over a 24-hour period, won't put your body into starvation mode. It doesn't happen that quickly and you are not depriving your body of vital nutrition.

Fasting Causes Overeating

This is a big one, and a slippery slope, when it comes to intermittent fasting. While your body is adjusting to the fasting lifestyle, it may be tempting to overeat when you break your fast and during a fresh eating window. This is only an initial potential pitfall while your body learns to adjust to your new eating schedule. Once it has become accustomed to your new lifestyle, the desire to and risk of overeating decreases dramatically.

For this reason, discipline, a healthy diet, and calorie consciousness are essential when you start intermittent fasting. Once you have adapted to fasting, you are no more at risk of overeating than if you were following a typical eating schedule.

Frequently Asked Questions

The content in the previous chapters has explained much of what you need to know about intermittent fasting and has probably answered most of your questions already. However, you may still have a few questions that need answering. Let's tackle some of those questions you may have outstanding.

How Long and How Often Should You Fast?

How long and how often you fast are based on several factors:

- Personal preference
- Choice of fasting plan
- Weight loss goals
- Lifestyle
- Gender
- Current health

The frequency of your fasting will depend on the type of intermittent fasting plan you choose to follow. You don't have to choose the most severe or even the most popular method. It comes down to a method that works for you personally and fits in with your lifestyle.

Your gender and weight loss goals also play a part in the decision of how long and frequently to fast. Some intermittent fasting methods, like the Fast 800 three-phase plan, are aimed at rapid initial weight loss to meet your goals before evening out into a maintenance phase that can be continued indefinitely. Other methods are aimed at slower weight loss through a fasting plan that can be maintained in the long term. Men may find it easier to fast for longer periods of time, while women often achieve better results with shorter fasting periods.

Your current health is a serious consideration when deciding on how long and frequently to fast and indeed whether or not to begin fasting at all. If your health is currently poor, it may be worth waiting and getting your overall health to a better level before starting a fasting plan. Yes, intermittent fasting offers a host of health benefits, but beginning a fasting plan when you aren't healthy could cause your health to deteriorate instead of improve. Always get approval from your family doctor before you start intermittent fasting.

As you can see, there is no right or wrong answer to this question and there isn't a definitive answer that will apply to everybody who wants to start fasting. A variety of personal individual parameters need to be taken into account to offer you the answer that best suits your own needs and body.

What Will Break Your Fast?

There is much debate about this question. Some intermittent fasting practitioners believe that only water should be consumed during a fasting period. Others say that a small, low-calorie, low-carb snack of less than 50 calories should be fine and not take your body out of a fasted state. There is no conclusive answer to this question, as both opinions are viable.

What about drinks? Hydration is an incredibly important part of any healthy diet. Your body is made up of over 70% water. Staying hydrated also makes fasting easier and helps your body to burn fat. Water is the obvious suggestion for hydration during your fasting period, but it's not the only option on the table.

Artificially sweetened beverages and the use of non-nutritive sweeteners, such as monk fruit, are allowed. They don't contain calories or carbohydrates which could inadvertently break your fast. These beverages include:

- black coffee or tea served without milk, cream, or creamer
- zero-calorie or zero-sugar carbonated beverages
- sugar-free sport and energy drinks

We know what you're going to say: "What if I hate black tea and coffee?" There is a way to get around not putting cream, milk, or creamer into your coffee and tea. These three traditional additions to coffee and tea introduce carbohydrates into your beverage, and risk taking your body out of a fasted state. You can swap them out for healthy fats such as a small amount of butter or even coconut oil.

These forms of healthy fats don't take your body out of a fasted state, or a state of ketosis. When it comes to intermittent fasting, it's not just about a zero-calorie intake while fasting. An integral part of the success of intermittent fasting is ketosis. Healthy fats like coconut oil and butter don't contain much in the way of carbs and therefore, won't kick your body out of ketosis.

Important note: Research into the effects of artificial sweeteners is ongoing. There are suggestions that artificial sweeteners may be bad for your health and some may cause side effects such as stomach upset. An alternative to artificial sweeteners is to use natural non-nutritive sweeteners which are derived from plants or alcohol sugars.

WEIGHT LOSS PROGRESS TRACKING

Transforming your body and your life by adopting an intermittent fasting lifestyle, eating a healthy diet, and walking as a form of regular exercise requires you to track your progress to measure your fat loss. Being able to measure your weight loss progress is an important motivator to keep you on track, determined, and committed to following through with such a significant lifestyle change.

Most of us turn to regular bathroom scales for the job, but they don't provide a true reflection of how much fat you are losing. If you are building lean muscle and burning off excess body fat at the same time, the number on the scale may appear to stubbornly refuse to budge, or even, much to your horror, sometimes go up. This is due to the fact that muscle weighs more than fat. If you are building a similar weight in lean muscle as you are losing in fat, the scale won't reflect any change. If you are building more lean muscle weight than you are losing fat, the number on the scale will even go up, which can be extremely discouraging.

There are better and more reliable ways of tracking your weight loss progress, which include:

- Body fat measurement tools, such as body fat scales and calipers
- The fit of your clothing, whether it is getting looser, and how much looser it is fitting over time
- A measuring tape to take body measurements such as hips, waist, chest, upper arms, thighs, and even calves. Loss of subcutaneous fat (the fat under your skin) will result in shrinking measurements

THE BOTTOM LINE

Intermittent fasting is a huge lifestyle change. It requires you to challenge and change the way you think and to develop mental resilience to face the challenges, rise to them, and conquer making such a considerable change. It also helps to bust some myths, answer some questions, and get some helpful tips and tricks to make the transition easier.

Overall, intermittent fasting is a lifestyle change that will transform your body, health, and life for the better. In the words of Frank Lloyd Wright, "You have to go wholeheartedly into anything in order to achieve anything worth having."

Your health and happiness are worth having. Intermittent fasting will help you to achieve them. It's just going to take a wholehearted approach and some work to make it happen, but it will happen.

HEALTHY LIVING BONUS

Guess what? We have included some further handy material to help you create a holistically healthy lifestyle. In the next chapter, we'll explore walking as the perfect exercise for anyone, any time, and explain why and how it compliments intermittent fasting so well that they create a weight loss power couple.

Walking is an amazing exercise that is entirely underrated. To sweeten the deal even more, we've added another bonus chapter (Chapter 7) on bodyweight exercise to help you build strength and lean muscle for a faster metabolism and healthy aging. Keep reading to find out how walking and bodyweight exercise can transform your body and your life!

PART II

BONUS: EASY EXERCISES TO BOOST YOUR FASTING

6

WALKING TO A SLIMMER, FITTER, AND HEALTHIER YOU

When you think about exercise, what comes to mind? Doubtless, the word evokes visions of sweating it out on a treadmill in a gym and feelings of physical, and even emotional, discomfort. You may even think of sports like football and tennis.

Walking is probably the last thing that will come to mind when you think about exercise. Walking is the unsung hero of the exercise world. It is the single most suitable and effective form of exercise for anybody and everybody. Sit tight because we're about to change your perception of walking for fitness and tell you how and why it complements the intermittent fasting lifestyle so well.

To help prove our point, let's define exercise.

> *"Bodily or mental exertion, especially for the sake of training or improvement of health: Walking is good exercise."*
>
> (Dictionary.com. (n.d.). Exercise.)

As you can see, even the dictionary agrees that walking is good exercise!

Having defined exercise as exerting yourself either mentally or physically, with the goal of improving health and fitness, walking fits perfectly into the category of exercise. In fact, according to Harvard Health Publishing of Harvard Medical School in the United States and the NHS in the United Kingdom, walking is one of the best exercises you can possibly do in terms of being low impact while still offering many health benefits.

WALKING VERSUS RUNNING

Now, you may be wondering how and why walking is so good for you compared to the likes of running, often considered to be the ultimate form of cardiovascular exercise. While there are some truths about running being excellent cardio, most people don't know the facts and therefore underestimate the power of walking.

Did you know that brisk walking (walking faster than you normally would up to a max of 4.5 mph) lowers your risk of high cholesterol, diabetes, and high blood pressure just as much as running does? That's right. The American Heart Association reported on research conducted among 48,000 walkers and runners. Among the participants in the study, it was discovered that mile for mile, running and brisk walking shared the same health benefits.

That being said, running does make your body work harder and therefore it does ramp up the cardiovascular intensity, but that isn't the be-all and end-all of exercise. What you're after are the holistic benefits of walking for weight loss and improved health, not just the intensity of exertion. The major distinction between walking and running is the duration. For a similar calorie burn and health benefits, it takes longer to walk the same distance than to run it. So, running will get you to where you want to be in half the time of brisk walking, but what's the catch?

The reason many people choose walking over running is that it's a gentler exercise that is suitable for a much larger percentage of the general population. Simply put, running puts a lot of stress on your body and comes with a much higher risk of injury. The stresses placed on your respiratory and cardiovascular systems, bones, and joints is significant, making it unsuitable for some people. This includes people with previous injuries, older individuals, and those with various health concerns, such as pre-existing heart disease or high blood pressure. Running puts you at a substantially higher risk of sprains, strains, fractures, and other impact-related injuries, even if you are healthy and just want to lose a few pounds.

While walking, you always have one foot on the ground. While running, you have what is known as "hang times," where you are completely airborne with both feet off the ground. The nature of gravity is such that what goes up must inevitably come down again. After that brief hang time, your foot must make contact with the ground to launch you into your next stride. This impact between strides places an immense amount of stress on your body, specifically your lower body and legs.

With each impact, your foot is striking the ground with the equivalent of roughly three times your body weight. For a typical runner of average weight, this translates to their legs absorbing over 100 tons of force from impact per each mile they run. That's a lot of impact force and it's that force that increases the risk of injury to between 20% and 70%, compared to between only 1% and 5% for walkers. If you do have joint concerns and are worried about the impact of walking, consult your physician for advice. You could also try using walking poles to improve balance, create a good rhythm, and help stabilise your body and joints at the same time.

WHY CHOOSE WALKING?

Aside from the much lower risk of injury we've just explained while comparing walking to running, there are other reasons to choose walking as your preferred form of exercise.

Weight Loss

Walking is the perfect exercise to help you shed unwanted pounds to transform your body and health for a slimmer, fitter, happier you. There are several ways in which walking helps you achieve your weight loss goals:

- Boosts your metabolism to increase your calorie burn during and after the exercise
- Improves the development of your lean muscle mass which burns more calories than fat by increasing your metabolism
- Improves the reduction in abdominal fat, reducing the risk of diseases associated with larger amounts of belly fat such as heart disease
- Including intervals and other body weight exercises in your walking improves post-walk calorie burn

Just About Anyone Can Walk for Health and Fitness

Although running is a popular type of cardiovascular exercise for weight loss and improved health and fitness, it is not suitable for everyone. You don't have to be older to experience trouble with running as exercise. Irrespective of age or gender, running is not always possible due to the amount of stress it places on your body. Individuals who cannot run as a form of exercise include:

- Those with medical conditions, such as heart disease and high blood pressure
- People who suffer from bone and joint diseases, such as arthritis
- People with previous injuries to bones, joints, and muscles
- Asthma sufferers
- Those on some forms of medication that can make strenuous physical activity problematic

These are just a few examples of people who cannot use running as exercise. These people would benefit greatly from adding walking to their lifestyle as a form of physical activity that promotes weight loss and improves health. Walking is gentle enough that anybody from toddlers to those in their golden years, people with existing medical conditions, pregnant women, those recovering from injuries, and many more can do it safely and comfortably.

The Perfect Beginner Exercise

Newcomers to the world of exercise may find the intensity and exertion of more strenuous exercise to be daunting even to think about. Society has conditioned us to believe that unless you're huffing and puffing, sweating profusely, and pushing your body to the absolute limit, you're not really exercising. This is entirely untrue and a myth that many beginner exercisers labor under and that ultimately leads them to give up, because the exercise is too intense, too quickly.

Walking, on the other hand, is the perfect way to ease into exercise. It is the perfect base upon which to build a physically active lifestyle, conditioning you for other exercises you may want to include once your initial fitness goals are achieved. It's gentle and it's a natural movement; you do it every day already, probably without even thinking about it.

Accessibility

Not only are the majority of people physically capable of walking, anyone who can walk for fitness always has access to it. No gym membership or expensive equipment is required. Walking requires very little equipment at all. The only basic requirements for starting a walking program are comfortable clothing, properly fitting walking shoes, and a healthy dose of motivation.

Health Benefits

Intermittent fasting and following a healthy diet already bring with them a host of health benefits. Walking offers many of the same benefits and thus amplifies the impact of each of the benefits you're already receiving. The health benefits of walking include:

- Improved cholesterol
- Improved cardiovascular health, and the risk of heart disease is reduced
- Improved blood pressure and a lowered risk of hypertension
- Lowered risk of diabetes
- Improved respiratory fitness
- Decreased risk of stroke
- Stronger muscles and bones
- Better balance
- Increased stamina and endurance

HOW WALKING AND INTERMITTENT FASTING WORK TOGETHER

Getting into the intermittent fasting lifestyle takes dedication, discipline, and work. It also takes some getting used to as your body adjusts from a typical eating pattern to a cyclic fasting schedule. This, in itself, may lead to some fluctuations in your energy levels as you go about your day-to-day life until your body has fully adjusted.

Adopting a physically active lifestyle is challenging in its own right. It's recommended to start out small and slow and work your way up to longer, more intense exercise sessions to allow your body to gradually become accustomed to exercise. Regular exercise has been shown to boost overall energy levels, but like fasting, your body will need to adjust to your new active lifestyle before the benefits of increased energy kick in.

Retraining your body to adapt to a new eating schedule and adding intense exercise at the same time may mean that you're setting yourself up for disaster and potentially giving up both intermittent fasting and an active lifestyle altogether. The key is to start off slowly with both fasting and exercise. Don't just jump into the most intense fasting plan and try to sweat it out at a high intensity every day.

Walking is a gentle, yet effective, exercise that is suitable for virtually everybody, carries a very low risk of injury, and is sustainable as a long-term exercise plan. When starting out in the fasting lifestyle, gentle exercise is encouraged as your body is placed under stress during the adjustment period. Walking is gentle enough that it doesn't place your body under much additional stress, thus allowing you to include physical activity from the start.

The efficacy of walking and intermittent fasting for weight loss and the fact that they complement each other so perfectly makes them ideal partners for adopting a healthy, active lifestyle.

MANPO-KEI (10,000 STEPS)

Have you heard about the 10,000 steps per day goal? It's a trend that began back in the 1960s. As Japan prepared to host the 1964 Tokyo Olympics, public awareness of the growing problem of preventable lifestyle-related diseases resulting from a sedentary modern lifestyle grew. Coincidentally, basic modern pedometers made an appearance and offered people a simple and practical way to track their daily activity and motivation to improve their basic fitness. It was during this time that the concept of manpo-kei was born.

Translated into English, manpo-kei means 10,000 steps. It became the motivational slogan for walkers who were dedicated to increasing their daily steps in a bid to improve fitness. A minimum target of 10,000 steps per day took root and has since continued to thrive as a daily step goal for walkers and the fitness conscious.

Does 10,000 steps a day really work, though? The School of Human Movement Studies at Queensland University and the Belgian Ghent University collaborated to find the answer to that question. In 2005 and 2006, a study was conducted to assess whether there were any provable grounds for manpo-kei or a 10,000 step daily target (Lashkari, 2016). A variety of participants were recruited for the study, ranging from people wanting to up their fitness to those who were predisposed to be at greater risk of developing lifestyle-related diseases such as cardiovascular disease. The findings reflected an improved sense of well-being reported among all study participants who managed to reach their daily 10,000-step goal.

Why Is 10,000 Steps Useful?

Considering the positive findings of the 2005 to 2006 study, 10,000 steps per day may help to improve your overall health and fitness and even help you to burn off extra weight. It is a useful and practical method for increasing fitness and improving health in a way that is simple, measurable and achievable.

You can easily track your daily steps by using a basic pedometer, an app on your smartphone, or a fitness watch. Tracking your steps for about a week before you begin trying to make your way toward manpo-kei provides you with a baseline or an idea of the average number of steps you take per day. Once that baseline has been established, you can then work toward gradually increasing your daily steps until you are achieving the minimum 10,000 steps per day.

WALKING OUTDOORS

The most natural place to walk is outdoors. Not only does the outdoors offer you plenty of space, but it also brings with it various benefits over walking indoors.

The benefits of taking a walk outdoors include:

- Fresh air: fresh air provides you with more oxygen than you find circulating indoors, which promotes better brain function.

- Stress reduction: getting outdoors and breathing in some fresh air boosts your mood by prompting your body to release endorphins, your natural feel-good chemicals, for improved mental and emotional well-being.
- Vitamin D: your skin needs direct exposure to sunlight to produce vitamin D, which is essential for a healthy brain.

Hiking

The idea of walking outdoors is typically synonymous with hiking. This type of outdoor walking puts you directly in contact with nature for the maximum feel-good effect. There is a lot of variability in hiking trails, making hiking suitable for beginners as well as the more advanced hikers, depending on which trails you decide to take.

Hiking ramps up your calorie burn and muscle conditioning, because it is more physically demanding than taking a walk in a city park or around your neighborhood. The varying terrain offers more challenges than simply walking on a flat and level surface, such as a street or a treadmill. Different types of terrain, from hard, rocky mountainside to soft, sandy beaches present unique challenges to different muscle groups for a more holistic walking workout.

Nordic or Pole Walking

Nordic walking employs the use of poles and arm swinging, which help you to speed up the pace and tackle uneven surfaces and inclines with better balance. The use of specialized walking poles brings your upper body into play more than regular walking, as you use your arms to plant the walking poles into the ground and thrust yourself forward.

Chi Walking

Chi walking engages your mind in a form of mindfulness movement meditation. Movements are controlled while you focus on the sensations of your body to achieve proper posture, bodily alignment, and walking form. Other areas of concentration include engaging your core muscles and connecting your entire being – body, mind, and spirit.

WALKING INDOORS

When the weather turns sour, you don't have to skip your walking workout. Taking your walking indoors helps you to get your steps in, irrespective of the weather. There are several options for walking indoors, not all of which call for access to a treadmill.

Treadmills

Treadmills aren't just for running. They are handy for walking indoors on days when the weather isn't conducive to getting outdoors. If you have the space available and can fit a treadmill into your budget, it's a great option.

Malls

Malls aren't only for window shopping and picking up essentials. They can be a great place to get your steps in. Depending on how busy the mall is, you can alternate between a slower pace in crowded areas and a brisk pace in areas where you can easily navigate around people and obstacles.

Indoor Tracks

Some health clubs and exercise facilities offer the option of indoor walking or running tracks which offer lanes for different walking speeds without obstacles or distractions. If you live or work close to an indoor track, it may be a viable option to get a dedicated walking workout in.

WALKING PACES

Some walking paces are best practiced outdoors where you have space to swing your arms and the ability to maintain the pace without having to navigate too many obstacles. Wide pavements or sidewalks provide the ideal environment to move around people and obstacles without having to slow down, breaking your rhythm.

Brisk Walks

Your fitness level will determine the speed of your brisk walk. The fitter you are and the more toned and conditioned your muscles, the faster you can walk. Brisk walking elevates your heart rate more than slower paces, to increase cardiovascular and respiratory performance. It also increases your calorie burn for the same workout length compared to a slower pace, as you can cover a greater distance in the same space of time. The average pace for brisk walking is approximately 3.5 miles an hour or 100 steps per minute.

Power Walks

Power walking is a full-body walking workout. Not only are you working your legs, but vigorous arm swinging also engages your upper body. To swing your arms correctly, bend your elbows at 90 degrees and keep your arms close to your body. When swinging, your hand should not come up higher than your breastbone. Your hands should also not come further across than the center of your body if you were to draw a line between the middle of your chest and your belly button. The average pace of power walking is between four and 5.5 miles an hour.

THE BOTTOM LINE

Walking is a simple yet effective form of exercise that is accessible to and suitable for the vast majority of people. It offers similar weight loss and health improvement benefits to running, without the high-impact and increased risk of injury that accompanies other, more intense forms of cardio.

Walking is a versatile workout that you can do indoors, outdoors, and at different paces to suit your needs. In the next chapter, we're going to take a look at how to maximize your walking workouts to get the most out of your exercise with useful tips and added exercises.

7

MAXIMIZE YOUR WALKING WORKOUT WITH THESE TIPS

There are two types of physical activity, or exercise, that adults need to participate in every week for holistic health and fitness. These physical activities will improve both your aerobic health – your cardiovascular system's ability to transport oxygen around your body – and your muscle strength.

The Centers for Disease Control and Prevention (CDC) is a respected health authority that has put time and research into how much exercise you should be getting every day or week. When you are new to exercise, it is important to acknowledge that you may not be able to immediately meet the CDC's recommended amounts of exercise for adults. That is okay; the important thing is to get started. Some physical exercise is preferable than none, and as you get fitter and stronger, you can work your way up to meeting, or even exceeding, the general recommendations.

The CDC offers some useful guidelines for how much exercise you should be getting to reap the health rewards of physical activity. Before we tell you how much exercise you should be getting per week, let's take a closer look at some types of exercises.

AEROBIC EXERCISE

Aerobic exercise refers to physical activity that gets your heart rate up and makes you breathe harder. This type of exercise is often referred to as cardio. The intensity of your physical activity refers to how much you are exerting yourself, or working, to perform that activity.

Moderate-intensity activities get your heart pumping and make you break a sweat. You should be able to have a breathy conversation, but not sing a song. Activities that count as moderate-intensity aerobic exercise include:

- Brisk walking
- Riding a bicycle on level ground with a small number of gentle hills
- Pushing a lawnmower

Vigorous-intensity aerobic activities increase your heart rate considerably and make you breathe hard enough that you cannot hold a conversation, but may be able to say a few words before you have to pause to take a breath. Activities that count as moderate-intensity aerobic exercise include:

- Running (6 mph or higher)
- Jogging (4 to 6 mph)
- Fast-paced bicycling or cycling on hills
- Playing sports such as football

MUSCLE-STRENGTHENING EXERCISE

Muscle-strengthening exercise refers to physical activity that strengthens and tones your muscles. Muscle strengthening exercises should work all of the major muscle groups, which are arms, shoulders, chest, back, abdominal muscles, back, hips, and legs. You should include muscle-strengthening exercises in your weekly workout routine for a holistic fitness program.

When performing this type of activity, specific movements target specific muscle groups. A complete movement from start to finish is referred to as a "repetition", or a "rep" for short. The number of repetitions you should aim for is between 8 and 12 at a time. Completing several reps before taking a short break is referred to as a set. For a complete workout of each muscle group, you should aim for two to three sets of each exercise per workout.

You can alternate between days on which you do cardio exercise or muscle-strengthening exercise, or you can do them on the same day. How you structure your weekly workout plan is entirely up to you and your schedule.

Activities that count as muscle-strengthening exercise include:

- Weight lifting
- Calisthenics or resistance body weight exercises such as squats
- Using resistance bands

HOW MUCH EXERCISE IS RECOMMENDED FOR ADULTS?

According to the recommendations of the CDC, this is the minimum amount of exercise an adult should be getting per week:

- Moderate-intensity aerobic exercise such as taking brisk walks: 150 minutes per week.
- Vigorous-intensity aerobic exercise such as jogging: 75 minutes per week.
- A combination of both moderate- and vigorous-intensity aerobic exercise such as intervals: alternating between moderate and vigorous-intensity in a workout on two or more days per week.

- Muscle-strengthening exercises: two or more days per week.

CROSS-TRAINING

Cross-training refers to including different types of aerobic and muscle-strengthening exercises in your workout program. Why is this important? It keeps your body on its toes when you switch things up, because your muscles need to adapt to different movements which work out different muscles.

An example of cross-training would be to switch up a walking routine with regular cycling. This teaches muscle groups to move differently, almost like your muscles learning new skills.

Cross-Training Benefits

Cross-training offers other benefits aside from preventing your body from adapting to a single routine which could stagnate strength and aerobic development.

Increased Muscle Fitness

Exercise can be seen as a positive form of stress on your body. The F.I.T.T. principle refers to the frequency, intensity, time, and type of exercise you perform. Coping with the same stress during each workout, day in and day out, allows your body to become accustomed to that particular type of stress, getting good at performing the activity. When your body is good at performing a specific activity, it makes exerting yourself more difficult because it gets easier for your body to handle.

Why would your body continue to work hard at increasing efficiency and fitness when it's already good at doing that exercise? Different types of exercise place different types of stress on your body, making it constantly adapt and work to become more efficient.

It Fires Up Your Metabolism

As we've just mentioned, when your body gets used to a particular exercise due to lack of variation in movement and the muscles worked, it hits a plateau and essentially stagnates. This leads to your metabolism doing the same thing. This is because you constantly use the same amount of energy when you perform the same movements to the same level of exertion. Cross-training makes your body use varying amounts of energy to work different muscles, so it fires up your metabolism instead of letting it stagnate.

It Keeps Things Interesting

People are creatures of habit, and they like routine and predictability. Once you have established a particular daily workout, you know the route or movements, how long it will take you to complete your workout, and how that specific workout will leave you feeling afterward. However, there is one problem with a lack of variation in your workout program.

Performing the exact same exercise routine day in and day out can get pretty boring. Boredom is a motivation killer. When you're bored with the same-old-same-old exercise, it's not fun anymore, you don't look forward to your workouts, and you lose motivation.

Cross-training keeps things interesting and can also increase overall satisfaction by offering you varied feelings of fulfilment, based on different levels of exertion and accomplishment.

It Decreases Your Risk of Injury

Performing the same exercise over and over each day indefinitely increases your risk of injury. This is especially true of high-impact or weight-bearing activities. You are subjecting the same bones, joints, and muscles to the same stresses all the time, not giving them a chance to rest properly while other muscles, bones, and joints get a turn to take the brunt of exercise stress. Eventually, fatigue can set in for these body parts, increasing your risk of both lesser and greater injuries.

HIGH-INTENSITY INTERVAL TRAINING (HIIT)

High-intensity interval training, has grown in popularity for the additional benefits it offers on top of the general benefits of exercise. It is a form of exercising that utilizes intervals. Your exercise alternates between short, sharp bursts of vigorous-intensity exercise with a recovery period of less intense exercise. It is important to note that interval training does not include rest periods where you stop moving to recover.

How long a HIIT workout session lasts isn't set in stone. There is no set duration, but because of the intensity of these workouts, they tend to last no more than 30 minutes. The length of the alternating intense and recovery periods is also not set. Traditionally, HIIT workouts use periods of 20 seconds of intense exercise and ten seconds for the recovery period. However, you can customize the length of these periods according to the particular exercises you are performing. For instance, if you are alternating between brisk walking and power walking, you could increase the intervals to three minutes of power walking and one to one and a half minutes of brisk walking. Another example would be alternating between three sets of body weight exercises and six minutes of brisk walking. The duration of the workout session also depends on the intensity of both the exercises you are alternating between.

The typical type of exercise used for intense periods is anaerobic exercise. Anaerobic exercise is not exactly the opposite of aerobic exercise. It doesn't lower your cardiovascular system's ability to transport oxygen to working muscles, but it doesn't improve it either. Often, the anaerobic exercise used in interval training is muscle-strengthening exercise, using weights or your own body weight to improve muscle tone and strength.

Benefits of High-Intensity Interval Training

So HIIT workouts increase the benefits of simply doing exercise, but they also offer additional benefits.

Increased Metabolic Burn

Human survival instinct is the reason high-intensity interval training is so effective at burning calories. Short bursts of intense energy output through physical exertion trigger a short-term metabolic rate increase in response to what your body interprets as a flight response to danger.

Why is this different from 30 minutes of brisk walking? Less intense activity sends a signal to your body that suggests you may be heading out on a long journey, possibly to find resources such as water and food. Your body then regulates your metabolism to conserve your energy reserves to cope with the potential of not finding those necessary resources for a while. Conserving energy for longer periods of travel helps you to survive when finding resources to replenish that energy isn't certain. On the other hand, conserving energy is your body's last concern when it perceives intense activity is a response to danger, and it's going to burn all the energy it needs to keep you alive.

Our modern living is a far cry from the time in our evolution when such automatic bodily responses to activity were a way of life. Our lifestyles have evolved much faster than our bodies and bodily functions. Therefore, you can use HIIT training to your advantage by tapping into that automatic energy-burning response to intense activity.

Lean Muscle Mass Increase

Lean muscle mass producing hormones are increased by short bursts of high-intensity physical activity. The increase in these hormones may be as much as 450% and the increase is sustained for a considerable period of time after performing the high-intensity activity. This increase in hormones promotes building lean muscle mass, which, in turn, aids weight loss by increasing your metabolic rate in response to more muscle consuming more energy.

Visceral Fat Reduction

Abdominal fat, or visceral fat, is the fat stored around your organs inside your abdomen. Visceral fat plays an important role in cushioning and protecting your organs, but too much fat in this area increases your risk of lifestyle-related diseases, such as:

- Heart disease
- High cholesterol
- High blood pressure or hypertension
- Type 2 diabetes
- Alzheimer disease
- Breast cancer
- Colorectal cancer

A short burst of high-intensity activity encourages your body to target this fat for burning.

Time Saving

High-intensity interval training burns more calories over a shorter period of time than exercising at a steady rate for longer. The UK's University of Aberdeen conducted a study that showed that five 30-second bursts of high-intensity activity with a four-minute recovery period afterward led to a three times greater fat burn than walking for 30 minutes at a steady pace (Walking for Health and Fitness, n.d.).

HOW TO TURN YOUR WALK INTO A HIGH-INTENSITY INTERVAL TRAINING WORKOUT

Turning your regular walking workout into a fat-burning, HIIT, cross-training session that will boost your weight loss and fitness is easier than you think. By adding body weight exercise to your walking routine, you can hit all the major muscle groups and reap even more rewards from your workouts, and here's how to do it.

- Set a timer for four minutes.
- Begin walking at a brisk pace.
- When the timer goes off and your four minutes are up, perform a set of body weight exercises for at least 30 seconds.

- Once your 30 seconds are up, begin walking at a brisk pace for another four minutes before performing another set of body weight exercises for 30 seconds.
- Repeat these walking and body weight exercise intervals throughout your walk.
- Aim to include three to four intervals when you first start. You can increase the number of intervals as your fitness and strength improve.

Tip: Choosing body weight exercises that you can perform anywhere and at any time is key to successfully incorporating calisthenics into your walks to create a HIIT cross-training workout.

Important note: We've previously said that a set of specific exercises should comprise eight to 12 repetitions of the exercise. When you start out, you may not be able to perform eight to 12 reps in the 30-second interval time frame. That's okay. Simply perform as many repetitions as you can without compromising form for speed. You will find you can perform more reps in the same space of time as your strength and fitness improve.

CALISTHENICS TO BOOST YOUR WALKING WORKOUT

Calisthenics are the ideal exercises to add to your walking routine. They require no special equipment, instead utilizing your own body weight for resistance. The following eight body weight power moves will help transform your body.

Important note: It may be tempting to try to squeeze as many repetitions of a body weight exercise into your 30-second interval period as you possibly can. When you are still learning to perform these exercises correctly, you should take it slow and pay special attention to your form while performing each move. Mastering the correct form before getting faster at doing the exercise is vital to properly work each muscle group and prevent injury. Correct form hits all the muscles intended for an exercise and allows you to do it safely. Poor form isn't as effective and could easily lead to injury such as strains, sprains, or worse. While performing each exercise, pay attention to how your muscles feel, your posture, and your breathing. Keep your core (abdominal) muscles tightened and engaged throughout the exercise.

Forward Lunges

Muscles worked: Quadriceps, glutes, hamstrings, hips

- Stand with your feet roughly six inches apart and your toes facing forward.
- Inhale as you take a step forward with your right leg, planting your right foot solidly on the ground.
- The heel of your left foot comes off the ground as you shift your weight onto the toes of your left foot and the whole of your right foot.

- Bend both knees to lower yourself toward the ground until both knees are bent to a 90-degree angle.
- Ensure that your right knee doesn't move forward past the toes of your right foot. Your lunge stride should be between two and 2.5 feet.
- The majority of your weight will be pushing down through the heel of your right foot with the toes of your left foot supporting only part of your weight and stabilizing your balance.
- Maintain a straight back and a tight core.
- Continue to maintain a straight back and a tight core. Exhale and push down through the heel of your right foot, using the toes of your left foot to stabilize yourself, to come upright and step back into the starting position.

You can perform all eight to 12 reps on the right side before switching to the left side for eight to 12 reps to complete the set or you can alternate, performing one rep on each side until you have completed the set. A set is only complete once you have performed the designated number of reps on each side.

Tip: Using a wider stride targets the glutes and hamstrings more, while a shorter stride works the quadriceps more.

Superman

Muscles worked: Lower back

- Lie on your stomach, legs straight and together.
- Extend your arms straight forward above your head on the ground.
- Maintain a neutral head and neck position. Don't tense your neck.
- Maintaining straight arms and legs, tighten your back muscles to raise your arms and legs toward the sky at the same time.
- Ensure that your knees and elbows are not locked.
- Your body should form a gentle curve, like a smile.
- Hold the Superman position for 30 seconds.
- Remember to breathe; it's tempting to hold your breath. Keep your breathing steady and rhythmic.

Tip: Don't try to over-arch your body in the beginning. Raise your arms and legs only as much as is comfortable. As your back muscles get stronger, you can lift your arms and legs higher. You can also switch things up a bit by holding the position for a shorter period and performing several reps to complete a set.

Skater Squats

Muscles worked: Quadriceps, hamstrings, glutes, outer thigh, hips

- Stand with your feet shoulder-width apart.
- Ensure that your back is straight.
- Straighten your legs but avoid locking your knees.

- Clasp your hands together in front of your chest, elbows bent.
- Inhale as you perform a squat by bending your knees, leaning forward from your hips, and pushing your butt out backward as if sitting down on a chair.
- Keep your core engaged, your back straight, and your chest up and out. Avoid rounding your shoulders.
- Squat as far as you can until your thighs are parallel to the ground. If you cannot squat that low to begin with, go only as low as is comfortable. You can always go lower as your strength and fitness increase.
- From the squatting position, exhale and push down through your heels, straightening up into a standing position.
- As you straighten up, shift your weight onto your right leg and extend your left leg out to the side with your toes facing forward.
- Inhale as you bring your left leg back into the starting position, feet shoulder-width apart, and spread your weight evenly between your left and right legs.
- Perform another squat by bending your knees, leaning forward from your hips, and pushing your butt out backward as if sitting down on a chair.

- From the squatting position, exhale and push down through your heels, straightening up into a standing position.
- As you straighten up, shift your weight onto your left leg and extend your right leg out to the side with your toes facing forward.
- Inhale as you bring your right leg back into the starting position, feet shoulder-width apart, and spread your weight evenly between your left and right legs.

This constitutes one full repetition of a skater squat. A repetition should not be regarded as simply performing a squat with only one leg extension to the left or right. Both legs should get a turn for it to be considered a single rep.

Tip: If you are having balance issues, you can use a nearby wall, lamp post, chair, park bench, or any other stable, solid support to help with your balance. You can also focus on a fixed spot to help with balance and improve concentration on mastering the correct form.

Triceps Dips (Bent Knees)

Muscles worked: Triceps

- Sit on the edge of a sturdy, stable bench, chair, low wall, or step. Sit up tall and straight to avoid slouching.

- Place your hands, palms down and fingers facing forward, on either side of your hips, and fold your fingers over the edge to get a good grip.
- Position your feet flat on the floor in front of you, slightly further forward than you would normally have them while sitting, and with your knees bent.
- Pressing down through your palms, lift yourself so that you are no longer sitting on the edge and shift slightly forward so that you are clear of the edge.
- You should now be suspended between your arms and feet. Keep your arms straight, but do not lock your elbows.
- Slowly bend your elbows to a 90-degree angle, lowering your hips toward the ground.
- Note that you shouldn't feel any pain in your shoulders and if you do, you are bending your elbows too much.
- Press down through your palms as you straighten your arms, raising yourself back up to the starting position in which you are suspended between your straight arms and feet.

Tip: As you progress and get stronger, you can increase the difficulty of the triceps dips by positioning your feet further and further forward. Once you are at a point where you can perform triceps dips with straight legs, remember to ensure that you do not lock your knees.

Pendulum

Muscles worked: Abdominals, oblique muscles down your sides, hips

- Lie on the ground on your back, legs straight and together, and your arms extended out to the side at a 90-degree angle to your body. Your body should form a T-shape.
- Raise your legs straight up, keeping your legs straight, but your knees shouldn't be locked.
- Keeping your legs together, exhale as you slowly lower your legs a few inches to the right.
- Don't allow your legs to go all the way over or touch the floor.
- Inhale as you raise your legs back to the center.
- Exhale as you lower your legs several inches to the left, again without lowering them too far over or letting them touch the ground.
- Make sure you keep your lower back in contact with the ground.

One rep consists of performing the pendulum motion to both the left and the right.

Calf Raises

Muscles worked: Calves

- Stand with your feet shoulder-width apart and your legs straight. Your knees shouldn't be locked.

- Ensure that your back is straight, shoulders relaxed, back, and down, and your chest us up.
- Exhale as you tighten your calf muscles and raise yourself up onto the balls of your feet.
- Hold this raised position for a count of two or three seconds.
- Inhale as you relax your calf muscles and lower yourself back down until your heels are just about touching the ground.
- Avoid allowing your heels to make full contact with or rest on the ground in between each raise repetition.

Tip: If you find you have trouble balancing while performing the calf raises, very lightly hold onto a wall, the back of a chair, a lamppost, or any other solid, stable object to help you keep your balance. Be sure not to rest more than your fingertips on the object; all you want to do is steady yourself, not use your hands to support your weight.

Plank

Muscles worked: Abdominals (core)

- Lie on your stomach on the ground, palms flat on the floor, next to your shoulders.
- Place your legs and feet together, extended straight with your toes facing downward and slightly tucked under you.

- Inhale as you raise yourself off the ground, pressing down through your palms.
- Lift your whole body off the ground as you straighten your arms.
- Your palms should be positioned almost right under your shoulders, balancing your weight between your palms and your toes.
- Keep the diagonal line of your body between your shoulders and toes as straight as possible without letting your hips dip or pushing them too high.
- Hold the plank position for 30 seconds and work your way up to holding it between one and three minutes as you get stronger and fitter.
- Remember to breathe throughout the exercise and keep your core engaged.
- Avoid shifting your weight from one arm to the other, keep it evenly spread between both arms.

Pushups

Muscles worked: Chest, shoulders, triceps

- Lie down on the ground on your stomach with your palms flat on the floor, positioned next to your shoulders.
- Place your legs and feet together, extended straight with your toes facing downward and slightly tucked under you.

- Inhale as you raise yourself off the ground, pressing down through your palms.
- Lift your whole body off the ground as you straighten your arms.
- Your palms should be positioned almost right under your shoulders, balancing your weight between your palms and your toes.
- Keep the diagonal line of your body between your shoulders and toes as straight as possible without letting your hips dip or pushing them too high.
- Inhale while bending your elbows to a 90-degree angle and lowering your chest toward the ground.
- Maintain a neutral position for your neck and spine.
- Exhale as you straighten your arms, pushing down through your palms to return to the starting position.
- When straightening your arms, don't lock your elbows.

This constitutes a single repetition. Aim for two sets of between ten and 12 reps.

IMPROVE YOUR ARM STRENGTH WHILE WALKING

Walking is a great leg workout, but your arms need the same amount of attention to build better upper body strength. HIIT walking workouts are fantastic for maximizing your calorie burn and conditioning your body through cross-training. However, you may not want to engage in HIIT walks every day of the week. There are a few tips and tricks for less intense walking workouts that you can use to get your arms involved.

Resistance Bands

Resistance bands are compact, light, and versatile for getting the most out of a walk. There are two types of resistance bands available; single length and continuous loop. A single-length resistance band is simply a long, straight piece of band that has two ends. A continuous loop resistance band is a circular band with no beginning and no end. Many trainers recommend the use of long single-length resistance bands with handles on each end over the use of continuous loop bands, as they are more versatile.

Triceps Resistance Band Exercise

- Behind your back, take hold of one handle on either end of the resistance band in each hand.
- Keep your left hand at your side while raising your right hand upward and bending your elbow so that your right hand is reaching down behind your right shoulder.
- From this position, straighten your right elbow, raising your right hand straight up into the air.
- Bend your right elbow, lowering your right hand to behind your right shoulder once again.

This constitutes one full repetition of the resistance band triceps exercise. Aim for performing two to three sets of between 12 and 15 reps per set. Repeat on the left side.

Light Weights

Light weights are useful additions to your walking workout equipment. You don't have to buy the most expensive weights and they will offer you a variety of arm-strengthening exercises to incorporate into your walks.

Light weights come in several forms. You can opt for hand weights, dumbbells, or wrist weights. Hand weights are self-explanatory. You are likely familiar with dumbbells. They are handheld weights that consist of a bar with either a solid weight on either end or adjustable plates that can be added or removed to increase or decrease the weight of the dumbbells as required. Wrist weights are essentially a band filled with sand or another weighted material that fit around your wrists. Most often, the closure is made of Velcro so the weights are adjustable to snugly fit your wrists.

There are a few differences between using wrist weights and handheld dumbbells while walking. The first difference is convenience. Wrist weights simply strap on around your wrists, leaving your hands free to be used for holding water bottles, answering a phone, or performing any other action while you're walking. When using handheld weights, your hands are holding on to the weights all the time, requiring you to stop and put them down if you want to use your hands for any other reason.

The second difference between wrist weights and dumbbells is the weight plates. Wrist weights come in set weight increments, requiring you to have several pairs of different weights if you want to increase or decrease the weight. When using adjustable dumbbells, you can simply loosen the fastener, slip a weight plate on or take it off, and screw the fastener back on. Each type of weight has its own advantages and disadvantages and the choice comes down to your personal preference.

The third difference is what you can do with the weights. Wrist weights are designed to be strapped on and don't offer much in the way of arm exercise versatility. You put them on, bend your elbows to 90-degree angles, and allow the wrist weights to work your biceps while swinging your arms. Using handheld weights, on the other hand, may not be as convenient as wrist weights. However, you can perform a variety of different exercises with them in addition to holding them in your hands, elbows bent to 90 degrees, and swinging your arms for a similar effect to wrist weights. These exercises include, but are not limited to, bicep curls, shoulder presses, overhead triceps presses, and lateral shoulder raises.

It's recommended to start off with a one-pound dumbbell or wrist weight. You can increase this weight to between two and five pounds as you build up your arm strength.

Important note: When using either dumbbells or wrist weights, there are a few precautions to take into consideration. Don't start off with a weight that is too heavy. You may think it's a light weight when you first pick it up, but carrying it around or performing various arm exercises with it while walking may be a different story altogether. While using weights during your walk, maintain the regular arc of your usual arm swing. Bend your elbows no more than 90 degrees (or less if you prefer) and keep your arms tucked close to your body. Avoid over-swinging your arms by swinging them too strongly or too high, as this can put your joints under pressure and cause strain, increasing your risk of injury.

Bench Exercises

Benches are often found along many popular urban walking routes. Of course, that depends entirely on where you walk. If your walking route includes a few benches along the way, an option for ramping up your arm strength is to utilize benches to perform isotonic body weight exercises.

Isotonic exercises keep constant tension on your muscles, making them work while moving. What this means is that, while performing the exercise, your body is in nearly constant motion and the tension in your muscles is also kept relatively constant. Isotonic exercise is the opposite of isometric exercise. To demonstrate the difference between them, take the following example:

Isotonic: performing push-ups keeps your muscles tensed to support your weight throughout the movement and your body is in near-constant movement, not stopping for any significant amount of time.

Isometric: performing a plank pose requires you to stay still while tension is kept on your muscles to hold your weight.

Every time you pass a bench during your walk, you can stop and perform a few simple arm exercises, such as push-ups using the seat rest or the backrest, and triceps dips. Please refer to the instructions on how to perform push-ups and triceps dips in the previous section on body weight exercises.

When using benches to incorporate arm-strengthening exercises into your walking routine, start with three benches and work your way up to include more benches as you get stronger. Aim to perform between ten and 12 reps of each exercise per set.

Isometric Exercises

As you've just learned, isometric exercises are the opposite of isotonic exercises. Isometric exercises keep tension in your muscles, making them work without movement. To perform isometric exercises, you hold a specific position for a set amount of time. A good example of an isometric exercise is the plank. Your body is held still in the plank position, making your muscles work to hold the position for the time period you set for yourself.

Chest Fly

- Press your palms together in the center of your chest, almost touching your chest.
- Press them together as hard as you can and hold for 20 seconds to perform one repetition.

Hands-Free Row

A hands-free row simulates a regular row done with a band or cable, and you can easily perform this exercise while walking or in a standing position.

- Extend your arms out in front of you and bring them back toward you, as if pulling a rower cable toward you.
- Pull your shoulders back, squeezing your shoulder blades together, and bend your elbows until they are in line with your waist or as far back as you can comfortably manage.
- When you have adopted this position, tighten the muscles on your arms and back as much as you can can and hold for 20 seconds to perform one repetition.
- Pay attention to your form to prevent yourself from pulling your shoulders upward into a shrug.

Bicep Curl

- With your arms at your sides, bend your elbows to bring your hands up to your shoulders as if performing a traditional bicep curl with a dumbbell.
- Tighten your bicep muscles as much as you can and hold for 20 seconds to perform one repetition.

Reps and Sets

When performing isometric arm exercises, aim to do between 10 and 15 reps per set and three to five sets per walking workout.

YOGA FOR TONING AND FLEXIBILITY

Yoga originated in ancient India has become a widely popular practice in modern fitness and health. Yoga makes use of controlled, deliberate movements that strengthen and tone muscles and increase flexibility. It is used as a form of exercise, for stress relief and relaxation, for mental health, and even spiritual well-being. It is not just a physical experience; it's meant to bring together and unify the body, mind, and spirit.

Yoga is a fantastic companion for fitness walking. It is more strenuous than tai chi, but less rigorous and has a lower impact than many other forms of exercise. There are several yoga poses that are perfect for walkers, helping to tone muscles and increase flexibility in all the right places to help prevent injury and increase range of movement.

Yoga Poses for Walkers

Forward Bend

Targeted areas: Lower back, hamstrings

- Stand upright with your feet shoulder-width apart.
- Take a deep breath as you raise your arms over your head. You can keep your hands straight or gently bend your wrists to create a slight arc. Your upper arms and ears should be in line.
- Lengthen your spine as if an invisible string is attached to the top of your head and is pulling you upward.
- Exhale deeply as you bend forward from the hips. Bring your arms down with you, keeping them in line with your ears.
- Once you have bent over forward as far as you can comfortably go, let your arms complete the downward journey so they come to rest, pointing downward, in front of your legs.
- Allow the muscles in your back and upper body to relax, bringing your chest toward your knees.
- Although your back muscles should be relaxed, avoid rounding or arching your back to force your chest toward your knees.

- Keep your shoulders relaxed to avoid shrugging them up to your ears.
- Hold the position for 20 measured breaths.
- To exit the posture, softly bend your knees and slowly roll your spine up, one vertebra at a time.

Tip: Never force your body into a stretch, as you could injure muscles. Only ever go as far into a stretch to allow you to feel the muscles stretching, but no pain. If you cannot reach your hands all the way to your ankles, bring your arms to your knees as you bend forward, supporting your upper body. You can slowly stretch lower as your muscles become more pliable over time.

Cat Pose

Targeted areas: Lower back

- Kneel on all fours on the ground.
- Position your hands directly below your shoulders, arms straight but elbows not locked.
- Position your knees directly below your hips.
- Inhale as you arch your back down toward the ground, and lift your chest and tailbone upward.
- Exhale while arching your back in the opposite direction, rounding it as you bring your chin toward your navel and tuck your tailbone forward under you.
- Repeat the stretch five times.

Tip: Perform the cat pose after every walk to help loosen the compression in your spine caused by walking upright.

Crescent Lunge

Targeted areas: Hip flexors

- Stand with your feet roughly six inches apart and your toes facing forward.
- Inhale as you take a step forward with your right leg, planting your right foot solidly on the ground.
- Bend your right knee, lowering your body toward the ground, until your knee is at a 90-degree angle.
- Ensure that your right knee doesn't move forward past the toes of your right foot. Your lunge stride should be between two and 2.5 feet.
- Keep your left, or back, leg straight, but don't lock your knee.
- Maintain a straight back and a tight core.
- Raise your arms straight upward above your head. You can keep your hands straight or gently bend your wrists to create a slight arc. Your upper arms and ears should be in line.
- Raise your arms from the shoulder, but be careful not to lift your shoulders upward into a shrug.
- Lengthen your spine as if an invisible string is attached to the top of your head and is pulling you upward.

- Tuck your tailbone in, pushing your hips slightly forward.
- Hold the position for 20 measured breaths.
- Repeat the pose on the other side.

Important note: If you cannot manage a full crescent lunge with your back leg extended straight, try placing the back knee gently on the floor and work your way up to performing a full lunge.

Plank Pose

Areas targeted: Upper body, core

- Lie down on your stomach, palms flat on the floor, next to your shoulders.
- Place your legs and feet together, extended straight with your toes facing downward and slightly tucked under you.
- Inhale as you raise yourself off the ground, pressing down through your palms.
- Lift your whole body off the ground as you straighten your arms.
- Your palms should be positioned almost right under your shoulders, balancing your weight between your palms and your toes.
- Keep the diagonal line of your body between your shoulders and toes as straight as possible without letting your hips dip or pushing them too high.

- Hold the plank pose for 20 measured breaths.
- Avoid shifting your weight from one arm to the other. Keep it evenly spread between both arms.
- Maintain a relaxed and straight neck while keeping your chest up and your head straight.
- Bring your knees to the ground and sit back on your calves, resting your chest on your knees or as low down to the ground as you can comfortably go.
- Relax your body with your arms outstretched on the ground in front of you.

Tip 1: If you cannot hold a plank pose or you feel your lower back is taking strain, lower your knees to the floor, maintaining the stretch in your upper body. Unlike kneeling on all fours, just lowering your knees to the ground without shifting them forward will cause your body to create a gentle upward curve from your feet to your head.

Tip 2: After performing a plank pose, bring your knees to the ground, shifting your weight back onto your heels while leaving your arms outstretched in front of you to stretch your upper back and shoulders.

Treadmill Walking Yoga Poses

Treadmills are a great option for indoor walking. They offer you much of the same physical exercise as you would get from walking outdoors. Your body will be moving in a similar way to walking on the pavement, so your muscles will be put under similar strain. You will need to warm and loosen them up before and cool them down after a treadmill walking workout. These yoga poses are ideal for treadmill walkers.

Side Plank

Areas targeted: Arms, core, wrists, upper body, balance

- Kneel on all fours on the ground.
- With your fingers spread wide, place your hands directly beneath your shoulders.
- Position your knees directly below your hips.
- Extend your right leg backward, turning your thigh upward for your inner thigh to be facing the sky. The bottom outside edge of your right foot will come to rest against the ground.
- Your body will twist as you perform the previous steps, positioning your left hip above your right hip.
- Your torso will also twist at this point until your chest is almost facing completely out to the side and you may not be able to keep your arms in their original position. As your torso twists, reposition your left arm closer to your chest for support.
- Rest your weight between your arms and your left outer foot while raising your right leg and lowering it on top of your left leg.
- At this point, your entire body, with the exception of the uppermost part of your torso, should be facing out to the side.

- Balancing your weight carefully between your left arm and left foot, raise your right hand off the floor and extend it toward the sky.
- Maintain a straight, diagonal line from your feet to your shoulders. Avoid allowing your hips to sag toward the ground.
- Hold the plank pose for between three and five deep breaths.
- Repeat on the other side.

Tip: If you have trouble performing the side plank, there are a few tricks to make it easier in the beginning. First, instead of using a fully extended arm to support the side plank pose, rest on your elbow instead, with your forearm on the ground at a 90-degree angle to your body. Instead of extending the non-supporting arm all the way upward, you can place that hand on your hip.

Dead Bug

Areas targeted: Hips, hamstrings, lower back

- Lie on your back on the ground, feet together and with legs extended.
- Bring your knees up to your chest, taking hold of the outside of each foot.
- Part your knees so your thighs rest along either side of your body, as parallel with your body as possible.

- Continuing to hold on to your feet, extend your lower legs upward toward the sky until your shins are perpendicular to, or at a right angle to, the ground.
- This pose opens the hips and stretches the hamstrings, releasing your lower back muscles.
- Hold the pose for ten measured breaths.
- After ten breaths, bring your knees closer together at your chest and do a gentle side-to-side rocking motion for a few moments.

Tip: If you find that you cannot grab hold of your feet, perform the pose without holding onto your feet and opt for extending your arms toward the sky. When doing this, your thighs should be as close to parallel with your body as possible with your lower legs extended upward, perpendicular to the ground, and your arms also extended straight up from the ground.

CONCLUSION

As you can see from what we've taught you, weight loss is achievable and it doesn't have to feel like self-punishment. You really can shed the extra pounds you're unhappy carrying around and keep them off, maintaining a healthy weight. Intermittent fasting, teamed up with walking, is the answer, and now you know why and how to incorporate them into your lifestyle.

Intermittent fasting is a lifestyle, not a quick fix that only delivers short-term results. It is healthy, contrary to what you may have been taught growing up or what sceptics may say. You can master the mindset necessary to adopt the fasting lifestyle and we've told you how to do it. We've provided you with all the information you need to switch to a healthy diet and start practicing intermittent fasting. You now know why walking is so effective and how to maximize

CONCLUSION

the benefits by switching things up with HIIT walking workouts, body weight exercises, and minimal equipment.

We've imparted a wealth of knowledge necessary to make positive lifestyle changes that are sustainable long-term. You know what you need to do to transform your life, lose weight, keep it off, get fit, and improve your health. Now all you have to do is take action and make it happen.

What are you waiting for? You have the power to take charge, make that transformation happen, and embrace health and happiness. Get fasting and get walking; there is no better time than right now.

A Free Bonus To Our Readers

To get you started on your intermittent fasting journey, we have created

- 40 Low-Carb Recipes
- 35 Mediterranean Recipes
- 35 Keto Recipes
- A 31-Day Meal Plan

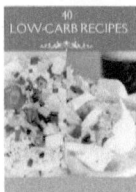 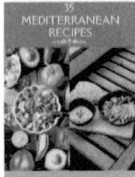 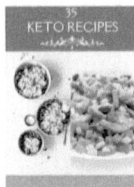 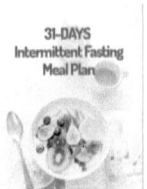

Free Bonus #1   Free Bonus #2   Free Bonus #3   Free Bonus #4

These 110 intermittent fasting recipes are delicious, healthy and easy to prepare. Each recipe includes serving sizes, nutritional data, and detailed step-by-step instructions. A weekly grocery shopping list is also included with the 31-Day Meal Plan.

To get your free bonuses, please click on the link or scan the QR code below and let us know the email address to send it to.

https://healthfitpublishing.com/bonus/iffw/

REFERENCES

Altmann, G. (2019, April 4). Question question mark questions symbol response. Pixabay. https://pixabay.com/illustrations/question-question-mark-questions-4101953/

Andry_Braynsk. (2020, May 8). Woman fitness girl beauty photoshoot hair legs. Pixabay. https://pixabay.com/photos/woman-fitness-girl-beauty-5140617/

Anne, R. (2018, October 1). Bye Bye Bat Wing 🦇 - TheQueenBuzz. Medium. https://thequeenbuzz.com/bye-bye-bat-wing-c336b332deac

Arps, Brianna. (2017, April 13). 9 psychological ways to help you lose weight. Independent. https://www.independent.co.uk/life-style/9-psychological-ways-weight-loss-easy-mind-strategies-every-day-a7682616.html

REFERENCES

B. (2019, February 7). Tim Spector: Breakfast—the most important meal of the day? The BMJ. https://blogs.bmj.com/bmj/2019/01/30/tim-spector-breakfast-the-most-important-meal-of-the-day/

Bacharach, E. (2019, November 18). 12 fasting tips that'll help you actually lose weight (and not go crazy). Women's Health. https://www.womenshealthmag.com/weight-loss/a29602869/fasting-tips/

Bailey, A. (2020, November 1). 5:2 diet meal plans: What to eat for 500 calorie fast days. Good to Know. https://www.goodto.com/food/5-2-diet-meal-plans-what-to-eat-for-500-calorie-fast-days-108045

Bendix, A. (2019, July 26). 8 signs your intermittent fasting diet has become unsafe or unhealthy. Insider. https://www.businessinsider.com/signs-intermittent-fasting-unsafe-unhealthy-2019-7?IR=T

Benefits of exercise. (2017, August 30). Medline Plus. https://medlineplus.gov/benefitsofexercise.html

Bjarnadottir, A. (2020, May 31). The beginner's guide to the 5:2 diet. Healthline. https://www.healthline.com/nutrition/the-5-2-diet-guide

Bob. (2020, August). Weight loss benefits of interval walking. Walking for Health and Fitness. https://www.walkingforhealthandfitness.com/blog/weight-loss-benefits-of-interval-walking

REFERENCES

Boone, T. (2007, December 4). Benefits of walking. How Stuff Works. https://health.howstuffworks.com/wellness/diet-fitness/exercise/benefits-of-walking.htm

Boyers, L. (3030, June 37). How to reach your daily step golas when working from home. Health and Wellness. https://www.cnet.com/health/how-to-reach-your-daily-step-goals-when-working-from-home/

Boyle Wheeler, R. (2017, May 4). Walking vs. running – Which is better? WebMD. https://www.webmd.com/fitness-exercise/news/20170504/walking-vs-running----which-is-better

Brenner-Roach, T. (2018, October 31). The 10 best intermittent fasting tips and tricks. Lift Learn Grow. https://www.liftlearngrow.com/blog-page/best-intermittent-fasting-tips

Bumgardner, W. (2019, June 24). How to start walking for weight loss. Verywell Fit. https://www.verywellfit.com/how-to-walk-for-beginners-3432464

Bumgardner, W. (2020, November 20). 6 best ways to take your walking indoors. Verywell Fit. https://www.verywellfit.com/best-ways-to-take-your-walking-indoors-3436836

Bumgardner, W. (2020, November 29). Tracking your walks. Verywell Fit. https://www.verywellfit.com/tracking-your-walks-3432825

REFERENCES

Carter, E. (2018, July 31). The benefits of adding cross training to your exercise routine. Michigan State University. https://www.canr.msu.edu/news/the_benefits_of_adding_cross_training_to_your_exercise_routine

Centers for Disease Control and Prevention. (2020, October 7). CDC. How much physical activity do adults need? https://www.cdc.gov/physicalactivity/basics/adults/index.htm

Chertoff, J. (2018, November 8). What are the benefits of walking? Healthline. https://www.healthline.com/health/benefits-of-walking

Clear, J. (2012, December 10). The beginner's guide to intermittent fasting. James Clear. https://jamesclear.com/the-beginners-guide-to-intermittent-fasting

Cottonbro. (2020, October 28). White and black menu board. Pexels. https://www.pexels.com/photo/white-and-black-menu-board-5723883/

Csatari, J. (2020, September 7). 6 mindset changes that help you lose weight fast, according to a celeb trainer. Eat This, Not That! https://www.eatthis.com/mindset-changes-lose-weight/

Discover Contributor. (2019, February 5). The dangers of intermittent fasting. Center for Discovery. https://centerfordiscovery.com/blog/the-dangers-of-intermittent-fasting/

Dolson, L. (2021, February 4). What is a whole foods diet? Verywell Fit. https://www.verywellfit.com/what-is-a-whole-foods-diet-2241974

Dr. Axe. (2019, April 4). Fasting? When it's time to eat again, here's what you should reach for first. The Upside by Vitacost. https://www.vitacost.com/blog/best-foods-to-break-a-fast/

Dreamypixel. (2017, August 11). Dolomites hiker landscape rock girl Italy hiking. Pixabay. https://pixabay.com/photos/dolomites-hiker-landscape-rock-2630274/

Dreyer, D. (n.d.). Build your core with chi walking. Active. https://www.active.com/fitness/articles/build-your-core-with-chi-walking?page=2

Eckelkamp, S. (2020, January 21). Intermittent fasting? Here's exactly what to eat at the end of your fast. Mind Body Green. https://www.mindbodygreen.com/articles/intermittent-fasting-heres-right-way-to-break-your-fast

Exercise and your arteries. (2019, June 21). Harvard Health Publishing Harvard Medical School.https://www.health.harvard.edu/heart-health/exercise-and-your-arteries

Fairytale, E. (2020, February 28). Women practicing yoga. Pexels. https://www.pexels.com/photo/women-practicing-yoga-3822169/

REFERENCES

Fairytale, E. (2020, February 28). Women practicing yoga. Pexels. https://www.pexels.com/photo/women-practicing-yoga-3822187/

Feinstein, K. (2020, June 1). Weight loss mindset: How to develop a mindset to lose weight. Red Mountain Weight Loss. https://www.redmountainweightloss.com/how-to-be-more-positive/

Fitday Editor. (n.d.). Understanding chi walking. Fitday. https://fitday.com/fitness-articles/fitness/cardio/understanding-chi-walking.html

5 signs you need a break from intermittent fasting. (2020, April 26). Slim Land. https://siimland.com/break-from-intermittent-fasting/

Foodnavigator.com. (2006, October 11). Americans recognize - but ignore - importance of breakfast, survey. https://www.foodnavigator.com/Article/2006/10/11/Americans-recognize-but-ignore-importance-of-breakfast-survey

Fotorech. (2018, June 20). Feet walk female feet young people walking ground. Pixabay. https://pixabay.com/photos/feet-walk-female-feet-young-3483426/

Free-Photos. (2016, March 21). Food meal soup dish peppers spicy stew healthy. Pixabay. https://pixabay.com/photos/food-meal-soup-dish-peppers-spicy-1209007/

REFERENCES

Giallo. (2018, February 8). Assorted silver-colored pocket watch lot selective focus photo. Pexels. https://www.pexels.com/photo/assorted-silver-colored-pocket-watch-lot-selective-focus-photo-859895/

Grady, M. (n.d.). Paraynama for pedestrians. Yoga International. https://yogainternational.com/article/view/pranayama-for-pedestrians

Good, C. (2017, January 18). 5 Fat Loss Myths (Unicorns)That Suck And What To Do Instead. Carter Good. https://cartergood.com/fat-loss-myths/

Gunnars, K. (2016, August 16). 10 evidence-based health benefits of intermittent fasting. Healthline. https://www.healthline.com/nutrition/10-health-benefits-of-intermittent-fasting

Gunnars, K. (2017, June 4). What is intermittent fasting? Explained in human terms. Healthline. https://www.healthline.com/nutrition/what-is-intermittent-fasting

Gunnars, K. (2019, July 22). 11 myths about fasting and meal frequency. Healthline. https://www.healthline.com/nutrition/11-myths-fasting-and-meal-frequency

Gunnars, K. (2020, April 20). Intermittent fasting 101 – The ultimate beginner's guide. Healthline. https://www.healthline.com/nutrition/intermittent-fasting-guide

REFERENCES

Gunnars, K. (2020, January 1). 6 popular ways to do intermittent fasting. Healthline. https://www.healthline.com/nutrition/6-ways-to-do-intermittent-fasting

Harris-Benedict equation by Wikipedia contributors. Wikipedia is licensed under CC BY-SA 4.0

Horton, B. (2019, April 2). Intermittent fasting the wrong way – Here's why. Cooking Light. https://www.cookinglight.com/eating-smart/nutrition-101/intermittent-fasting-mistakes

How fasting might make our cells more resilient to stress. IFL Science. https://www.iflscience.com/health-and-medicine/how-fasting-might-make-our-cells-more-resilient-stress/

How to start intermittent fasting in 5 non-intimidating steps. (2018, September 29). Mindful Keto. https://mindfulketo.com/how-to-start-fasting/

Intermittent fasting: What is it, and how does it work? John Hopkins Medicine. https://www.hopkinsmedicine.org/health/wellness-and-prevention/intermittent-fasting-what-is-it-and-how-does-it-work

Insulin resistance & prediabetes. (2019, March 3). National Institute of Diabetes and Digestive and Kidney Diseases. https://www.niddk.nih.gov/health-information/diabetes/overview/what-is-diabetes/prediabetes-insulin-resistance

REFERENCES

Intermittent fasting by Wikipedia contributors, Wikipedia is licensed under CC BY-SA 4.0

Jarreau, P. (2019, May 16). A beginner's guide to intermittent fasting. Life Apps. https://lifeapps.io/fasting/a-beginners-guide-to-intermittent-fasting/

Jerreau, P. (2020, May 18). The 5 stages of intermittent fasting. Life Apps. https://lifeapps.io/fasting/the-5-stages-of-intermittent-fasting/

Johnson, J. (2019, January 28). How to do the 5:2 diet. Medical News Today. https://www.medicalnewstoday.com/articles/324303

Kamb, S. (2021, January 1). Intermittent fasting beginner's guide (should you skip breakfast?) Nerd Fitness. https://www.nerdfitness.com/blog/a-beginners-guide-to-intermittent-fasting/

Kubala, J. (2020, January 7). Eat stop eat review: Does it work for weight loss? Healthline. https://www.healthline.com/nutrition/eat-stop-eat-review

Kwan, N. (2011, November 3). Yoga poses for walkers. Prevention. https://www.prevention.com/fitness/fitness-tips/a20478110/yoga-positions-to-improve-walking-workouts/

Lashkari, C. (2016, October 9. Where did 10,000 steps a day come from? News Medical. https://www.news-medical.net/health/Where-did-10000-steps-a-day-come-

REFERENCES

from.aspx

Lehman, S. (2020, November 22). How many calories do I need each day? Verywell Fit. https://www.verywellfit.com/how-many-calories-do-i-need-each-day-2506873

Leiva, C. (2018, October 10). The best and worst types of intermittent fasting, according to experts. Insider. https://www.insider.com/best-worst-intermittent-fasting-types-2018-9

Leonard, J. (2020, April 16). Seven Ways to do intermittent fasting. Medical News Today. https://www.medicalnewstoday.com/articles/322293

Leonard, J. (2020, January 17). A guide to 16":8 intermittent fasting. Medical News Today. https://www.medicalnewstoday.com/articles/327398

Lidicker, G. (2020, January 8). Intermittent fasting tips & tricks from experts. Chowhound. https://www.chowhound.com/food-news/251799/intermittent-fasting-tips-tricks/

Link, R. (2018, September 4). 16/8 intermittent fasting: A beginner's guide. Healthline. https://www.healthline.com/nutrition/16-8-intermittent-fasting

Lose weight, stay healthy, live longer. (n.d.). The Fast 800. https://thefast800.com/

REFERENCES

Lowery, M. (2017, September 18). Top 5 intermittent fasting mistakes. 2 Meal Day. https://2mealday.com/article/top-5-intermittent-fasting-mistakes/

Malacoff, J. (2020, January 17). 5 ways walkers can strengthen their arms. Myfitnesspal. https://blog.myfitnesspal.com/5-ways-walkers-can-strengthen-their-arms/

Marcin, A. (2018, March 5). 6 ways to measure body fat percentage. Healthline. https://www.healthline.com/health/how-to-measure-body-fat

Mayo Clinic Staff. (n.d.). Walking: Make it count with activity trackers. Mayo Clinic. https://www.mayoclinic.org/healthy-lifestyle/fitness/in-depth/walking/art-20047880

Mayoclinic Staff. (n.d.). Tai chi: A gentle way to fight stress. Mayoclinic. https://www.mayoclinic.org/healthy-lifestyle/stress-management/in-depth/tai-chi/art-20045184

Mediterranean diet. (n.d.). U.S. News and World Report. https://health.usnews.com/best-diet/mediterranean-diet

Melinda. (2019, March 20). Emotional eating and how to stop it. HelpGuide.org. https://www.helpguide.org/articles/diets/emotional-eating.htm

Melinda. (2019, March 20). Emotional eating and how to stop it. HelpGuide.org. https://www.helpguide.org/articles/diets/emotional-eating.htm

REFERENCES

Migala, J. (2018, July 25). The ultimate guide to following a low-carb diet: What to eat and avoid, a sample menu, health benefits and risks, and more. Everyday Health. https://www.everydayhealth.com/diet-nutrition/diet/low-carb-diet-beginners-guide-food-list-meal-plan-tips/

Migala, J. (2020, April 20). The 7 types of intermittent fasting, and what to know about them. Everyday Health. https://www.everydayhealth.com/diet-nutrition/diet/types-intermittent-fasting-which-best-you/

Miranda, J. (2020, March 29). Similar cubes with rules inscription on windowsill in building. Pexels. https://www.pexels.com/photo/similar-cubes-with-rules-inscription-on-windowsill-in-building-4027658/

Monstera. (2020, September 18). Multiethnic women practicing yoga in park. Pexels. https://www.pexels.com/photo/multiethnic-women-practicing-yoga-in-park-5384564/

Monstera. (2020. September 10). Anonymous woman stretching body in extended child s yoga pose. Pexels. https://www.pexels.com/photo/anonymous-woman-stretching-body-in-extended-child-s-yoga-pose-5331223/

Mueller, J. (2015, February 2). 8 strength training moves for walkers. Sparkpeople. https://www.sparkpeople.com/resource/fitness_articles.asp?id=2021

Olsson, E. (2018, November 27). Flat-lay photography of vegetable salad on plate. Pexels.

REFERENCES

https://www.pexels.com/photo/flat-lay-photography-of-vegetable-salad-on-plate-1640777/

Paravantes, E. (2019, June 27). The complete guide to the authentic Mediterranean diet. Olive Tomato. https://www.olivetomato.com/complete-guide-authentic-mediterranean-diet/

Paige, C. (2021, July 26). Almond Berry Crisp with Whipped Cream (Vegan & Gluten-Free Recipe). FitLiving Eats by Carly Paige. https://www.fitlivingeats.com/almond-berry-crisp-decadent-coconut-whipped-cream/

Pattillo, A. (n.d.). Intermittent fasting: A popular diet with serious psychological risks. Inverse. https://www.inverse.com/article/58082-intermittent-fasting-psychological-risks-binge-eating

Piacquadio, A. (2020, February 24). Flexible ethnic athlete doing standing forward bend exercise on street in city. Pexels. https://www.pexels.com/photo/flexible-ethnic-athlete-doing-standing-forward-bend-exercise-on-street-in-city-3799382/

Piacquadio, A. (2020, February, 20). Group of women doing exercise inside the building. Pexels. https://www.pexels.com/photo/group-of-women-doing-exercise-inside-the-building-3775566/

Pixabay. (2016, April 24). Black magnifying glass. Pexels. https://www.pexels.com/search/question/

REFERENCES

Rabbitt, M. (2020, July 15). 10 biggest benefits of walking to improve your health, according to experts. Prevention. https://www.prevention.com/fitness/a20485587/benefits-from-walking-every-day/

Rachelstallone, R. (2021b, July 27). Running vs. walking, which is actually better for you? Netherlands News Live. https://netherlandsnewslive.com/running-vs-walking-which-is-actually-better-for-you/207202/

Ramos, M. (2021, January 20). How to break your fast. Diet Doctor. https://www.dietdoctor.com/intermittent-fasting/how-to-break-your-fast

Ries, J. (2020, January 3). This is your body on intermittent fasting. Huff Post. https://www.huffpost.com/entry/body-intermittent-fasting_l_5e0a3220c5b6b5a713b22dcb

Ring, F. (n.d.). Weight loss benefits of interval walking – Increase your metabolism. Walking For Health And Fitness. https://www.walkingforhealthandfitness.com/blog/weight-loss-benefits-of-interval-walking

Robertson, K. (2017, March 7). 10 meal plan ideas for 6:2 fast days. Get The Gloss. https://www.getthegloss.com/article/10-days-of-meal-ideas-for-5-2-fasting-days

Rutledge, T. (2020, June 3). The psychology of intermittent fasting. Psychology Today. https://www.psychologytoday.com/za/blog/the-healthy-journey/202006/the-psychology-intermittent-fasting

Santilli, M. (2020, February 17). Everything you need to know before doing intermittent fasting while pregnant. Health 24. https://www.news24.com/health24/parenting/pregnancy/nutrition/everything-you-need-to-know-before-doing-intermittent-fasting-while-pregnant-20200217-2

Shepherd, D. (2018, October 23). What to expect when intermittent fasting: 11 experiences from 4+ years of IF. Hunger For Excellence. https://www.huffpost.com/entry/body-intermittent-fasting_l_5e0a3220c5b6b5a713b22dcb

Sikkema, K. (2020, March 20). Orange and black USB cable on brown wooden surface. Unsplash. https://unsplash.com/photos/IZOAOjvwhaM

Sinkus, T. (20201, January 9). A full beginner's guide to intermittent fasting + daily plan. 21 Day Hero. https://21-dayhero.com/intermittent-fasting-daily-plan/

Steinhilber, B. (2018, May 4). Why walking is the most underrated form of exercise. NBC News. https://www.nbcnews.com/better/health/why-walking-most-underrated-form-exercise-ncna797271

Stewart, T. (2018, May 15). Increase Your Flexibility This Summer With Core Stretches. Vitalize Magazine. https://vitalizemagazine.com/increase-your-flexibility-this-summer-with-core-stretches/

REFERENCES

Streit, L. (2019, December 12). The flexitarian diet: A detailed beginner's guide. Healthline. https://www.healthline.com/nutrition/flexitarian-diet-guide

Sweat. (2019, October 28). LowIntensity Cardio Training What Is It How Does It Work. https://www.sweat.com/blogs/fitness/low-intensity-cardio

Taub-Dix, B. (2019, January 3). What is a flexitarian diet? What to eat and how to follow the plan. https://www.everydayhealth.com/diet-nutrition/diet/flexitarian-diet-health-benefits-food-list-sample-menu-more/

TeeRifficU. (2020, April 21). Why 10,000 Steps Per Day? Manpo-Kei. . . That's Why! | teerifficu. https://teerifficu.com/why-10000-steps-per-day-manpo-kei-thats-why/

The Editors. (2021, February 9). Fasting. Britannica. https://www.britannica.com/topic/fasting

The insulin resistance – Diabetes connection. (2019, August 12). Centers for Disease Control and Prevention. https://www.cdc.gov/diabetes/basics/insulin-resistance.html

Thompson, Claudia. (2019, August 20). What to eat on your low-calorie days if you're doing a 5:2 fast. Livestrong. https://www.healthline.com/nutrition/how-to-fast

TotalShape. (2019, April 27). Weight loss fitness lose weight health workout. Pixabay. https://pixabay.com/illustrations/question-question-mark-questions-4101953/

REFERENCES

U.S. Department of Health and Human Services. (n.d.). Weight and obesity | Office on Women's Health. Office on Women's Health. https://www.womenshealth.gov/healthy-weight/weight-and-obesity

Van De Walle, G. (2019, December 12). What is a calorie deficit, and how much of one is healthy? Healthline. https://www.healthline.com/nutrition/calorie-deficit

Waehner, P. (2020, January 21). How to track your weight loss progress. Verywell Fit. https://www.verywellfit.com/ways-to-track-weight-loss-progress-1231581

Wave, M. (2021, January 10). Supportive woman doing plank in room. Pexels. https://www.pexels.com/photo/sportive-woman-doing-plank-in-room-6453942/

Weight loss: 5 ways to avoid overeating on intermittent fasting. (2020, April 15). Times of India. https://timesofindia.indiatimes.com/life-style/health-fitness/diet/weight-loss-5-ways-to-avoid-overeating-on-intermittent-fasting/photostory/75144887.cms

Weiner, Z. (2020, March 18). Why it's important to do stretches before walking, no matter how many steps you're clocking. Well And Good. https://www.wellandgood.com/stretches-before-walking/

West, H. (2019, January 2). How to fast safely: 10 helpful tips. Healthline. https://www.healthline.com/nutrition/how-to-fast

REFERENCES

Why warming up and cooling down is important. (2016, December 15). Tri-City Medical Center. https://www.tricitymed.org/2016/12/warming-cooling-important/

Wikipedia Contributors. (2018, December 7). Harris-Benedict equation. Wikipedia; Wikimedia Foundation. https://en.wikipedia.org/wiki/Harris%E2%80%93Benedict_equation

Wikipedia. (2021, June 16). Yoga. Wikipedia. Retrieved June 18, 2020, from https://en.wikipedia.org/wiki/Yoga

Williams, C. (2018, June 1). How intermittent fasting affects your metabolism. Cooking Light. https://www.cookinglight.com/healthy-living/healthy-habits/how-fasting-affects-metabolism

Wong, N. (2021, April 25). 5 types of diets and their benefits. MSN Lifestyle. https://www.msn.com/en-my/lifestyle/other/5-types-of-diets-and-their-benefits/ar-BB1g2rSQ

WorkoutLabs. (n.d.). Spin / Push Up Rotations – WorkoutLabs Exercise Guide. https://workoutlabs.com/exercise-guide/spin-push-up-rotations/

Yoshiki, K. (2016, September 21). Man push up on white floor. Pexels. https://www.pexels.com/photo/man-push-up-on-white-floor-176782/

LEAVE A REVIEW

If you enjoyed this book, please leave some feedback, even if it's just a few words!

Your feedback helps us to provide the best quality books and helps other readers like you, discover great books that they will also enjoy.

Please click on the link below or click/scan the QR code to leave feedback on Amazon.

https://www.amazon.com/review/create-review/?asin=

ALSO BY HEALTHFIT PUBLISHING

Walking Your Way to Weight Loss: A Simple Two-Part Approach to Becoming Fitter, Healthier, and Happier in 49 Days

Intermittent Fasting for Women: A Guide to Creating a Sustainable, Long-Term Lifestyle for Weight Loss and Better Health! Includes How to Start, 16:8, 5:2, OMAD, Fast 800, ADM, Warrior and Fast 5!

www.ingramcontent.com/pod-product-compliance
Lightning Source LLC
Chambersburg PA
CBHW022043160426
43209CB00002B/45